PSYCHOLOGICAL DISORDERS OF CHILDREN

McGraw-Hill
Series in Psychology

Consulting Editors
Norman Garmezy
Richard L. Solomon
Lyle V. Jones
Harold W. Stevenson

Hurlock   *Developmental Psychology*
Jackson and Messick   *Problems in Human Assessment*
Krech, Crutchfield, and Ballachey   *Individual in Society*
Lakin   *Interpersonal Encounter: Theory and Practice in Sensitivity Training*
Lawler   *Pay and Organizational Effectiveness: A Psychological View*
Lazarus, A.   *Behavior Therapy and Beyond*
Lazarus, R.   *Adjustment and Personality*
Lewin   *A Dynamic Theory of Personality*
Lewin   *Principles of Topological Psychology*
Maher   *Principles of Psychopathology*
Marascuilo   *Statistical Methods for Behavioral Science Research*
Marx and Hillix   *Systems and Theories in Psychology*
Miller   *Language and Communication*
Morgan   *Physiological Psychology*
Mulaik   *The Foundations of Factor Analysis*
Novick and Jackson   *Statistical Methods for Educational and Psychological Research*
Nunnally   *Psychometric Theory*
Overall and Klett   *Applied Multivariate Analysis*
Robinson and Robinson   *The Mentally Retarded Child*
Rosenthal   *Genetic Theory and Abnormal Behavior*
Ross   *Psychological Disorders of Children: A Behavioral Approach to Theory, Research, and Therapy*
Schwitzgebel and Kolb   *Changing Human Behavior: Principles of Planned Intervention*
Shaw   *Group Dynamics: The Psychology of Small Group Behavior*
Shaw and Costanzo   *Theories of Social Psychology*
Shaw and Wright   *Scales for the Measurement of Attitudes*
Sidowski   *Experimental Methods and Instrumentation in Psychology*
Siegel   *Nonparametric Statistics for the Behavioral Sciences*
Spencer and Kass   *Perspectives in Child Psychology*
Stagner   *Psychology of Personality*
Townsend   *Introduction to Experimental Methods for Psychology and the Social Sciences*
Vinacke   *The Psychology of Thinking*
Wallen   *Clinical Psychology: The Study of Persons*
Warren and Akert   *The Frontal Granular Cortex and Behavior*
Waters, Rethlingshafer, and Caldwell   *Principles of Comparative Psychology*
Winer   *Statistical Principles in Experimental Design*
Zubek and Solberg   *Human Development*

PSYCHO-LOGICAL DISORDERS OF CHILDREN

A BEHAVIORAL APPROACH TO THEORY, RESEARCH, AND THERAPY

ALAN O. ROSS

McGRAW-HILL BOOK COMPANY

New York   St. Louis   San Francisco   Düsseldorf   Johannesburg
Kuala Lumpur   London   Mexico   Montreal   New Delhi
Panama   Rio de Janeiro   Singapore   Sydney   Toronto

Library of Congress Cataloging in Publication Data

Ross, Alan O
    Psychological disorders of children.

    (McGraw-Hill series in psychology)
    Bibliography: p.
    1. Child psychiatry. I. Title.
[DNLM: 1. Behavior therapy—In infancy and
childhood. 2. Child behavior disorders.
3. Learning disorders.   4. Mental disorders—
In infancy and childhood. 5. Mental retardation.
WS350 R823   1974]
RJ 499.R66   618.9′28′9   73–6617
ISBN 0-07-053867-0

PSYCHOLOGICAL DISORDERS OF CHILDREN:
A Behavioral Approach to Theory, Research, and Therapy

1 2 3 4 5 6 7 8 9 0 K P K P 7 9 8 7 6 5 4 3

This book was set in Univers.
The editors were Walter Maytham and Phyllis Dulan;
the designer was Nicholas Krenitsky;
and the production supervisor was Ted Agrillo.
The printer and binder was Kingsport Press, Inc.

TO ILSE
- - for being

CONTENTS

ix

PREFACE

Clinical psychology is witnessing a resurgence of interest as knowledge about human behavior, based on laboratory experiments, is finding application in the study and treatment of psychological disorders. This has led to the appearance of several books which present the deviant behavior of adults from what has come to be called the behavioral point of view. At the same time, students who wish to explore the deviant behavior of children from this perspective have had to rely on journal articles and project reports or on texts written in the psychodynamic orientation. This book was written to fill the need for a behaviorally oriented presentation of psychological disorders of children and of their treatment through behavior therapy[1].

I have addressed myself to advanced undergraduates and to beginning graduate students in psychology and such related fields as social work, special education, and child psychiatry. In so doing, I have made the assumption that the reader has some background

[1] Since I consider psychology to be the science of behavior, I freely interchange the terms *psychological* and *behavioral*, speaking at one point about psychological, at another about behavioral disorders. The title of this book might thus just as easily have been Behavior Disorders of Children : A Psychological Approach.

in the behavioral sciences and familiarity with the principles of behavior as they are expressed in current theories of learning. Those wishing to review the principles essential for ready comprehension of the exposition to follow, may find it useful to turn to Chapter 12 before proceeding to Chapter 1.

The behavioral point of view, from which this book is written, is not the methodological behaviorism that categorically excludes from consideration any event that is not subject to direct observation. Nor have I limited myself to the formulations of operant conditioning, valuable though I find this approach to be. The behavioral orientation that guided my writing places a great deal of emphasis on the all-important role of the social environment in shaping and maintaining human behavior, but it also makes room for such concepts as self-control, self-observation, observational learning, and cognitive mediation as well as for a limited number of operationally defined constructs, such as anxiety and anger. Some readers may recognize this as the approach of social learning theorists and I gladly acknowledge the influence, not only of my own teachers, John Dollard and Neal Miller, but also of Albert Bandura and his students. Whatever my approach might be labeled, I hope that it reflects a firm commitment to hew as closely as possible to the data from available research.

In the field of psychological disorders of children, research-based knowledge is, unfortunately, more readily available in some topic areas than in others. As a result, the chapters of this book are of unequal length. Where, as on psychophysiological disorders, there is a dearth of data, there are few pages; where, as on aggressive behavior, there is a profusion of data, there are many pages. I chose not to compensate for a paucity of knowledge by the presentation of armchair speculations or colorful case histories. In most instances, the investigators whose work I discuss operate in a frame of reference that is cognate to my own. At times, however, as in the chapters on early infantile autism and juvenile delinquency, I have presented the theoretical formulations of authors who take a different approach. The justification for this is that these writers stay sufficiently close to research-based data that their ideas deserve a hearing, particularly since they may well have a seminal influence on further research.

Except in rare instances where clarity of exposition seemed to demand such reference or when my fractious nature overwhelmed my amicable intent, I have avoided the juxtaposition of the behavioral with the traditional, the so-called psychodynamic approach to the topic. With the bias I try to make explicit, I could but attack the psychodynamic approach without providing the reader the opportunity to see a reasoned rebuttal. Even if a rebuttal could have been provided, the superiority of one frame of reference over another is no more proved by argument than by polemic. The test must be the pragmatic one of which approach best integrates available facts and which best serves to generate effective methods for helping disturbed children and preventing disturbances in others. Definitive answers to these questions are not available, but as I have, over the years, tried first one approach and then the other, I have become persuaded of the superiority of the behavioral approach. In the final analysis, the choice of a theory is not a matter of truth but of judgment. I would hope that the scholarly reader will seek out one of the many fine expositions of alternate points of view and arrive at his own judgment.

In a sense, this book represents the payment of a debt. A few years ago (Ross, 1967b) I had occasion to review a book on child psychopathology, written by a highly regarded fellow psychologist. After recording some well-deserved commendations about this work, I wrote:

If clinical child psychology is to justify its existence it must make a unique contribution to the prevention and treatment of psychological disorders by bringing the knowledge of child psychology to bear on clinical problems. The last few years have seen an increasing awareness of the relevance of laboratory research to clinical practice and a concomitant, growing interest of the laboratory researcher in clinical problems. It is because this book ignores these developments that it is a disappointment despite its many positive qualities (p. 418).

Even as I wrote these lines, I heard a still small voice say "Let's see you do better," and so I set out to attempt a book on the psychological disorders of children that would, I hoped, succeed where I had accused my colleague of failing. I trust, in some ways, that I have redeemed the debt I incurred by voicing my reproof.

In preparing this book I had the much appreciated assistance of my daughter Judy, who spent a summer vacation searching out references and copying abstracts. The prompt, neat, and accurate clerical support provided by Socorro Watson was an important help for which I am most appreciative. While they do not share the prefatory inscription, my daughters, Judy and Pam, are assured of my affection as I reserve my most profound gratitude to my wife, Ilse Wallis Ross, to whom alone this book is dedicated. As together we traversed from the psychodynamic to the behavioral orientation, her abiding interest in people and her remarkable clinical acumen as a social worker have provided a needed and constructive foil to my enthusiasm for scientific objectivity.

ACKNOWLEDGMENTS

For granting me permission to quote from their writings, I am indebted to Drs. Wesley C. Becker, Lovick C. Miller, and Donald R. Peterson. Corporate holders of copyrights who permitted me to quote from their material and whose courtesy is hereby acknowledged are: Academic Press, American Association for the Advancement of Science, American Psychological Association, American Psychosomatic Association, Dorsey Press, Hoeber Medical Division of Harper and Row, McGraw-Hill Book Company, and The Society for Research in Child Development. Where requested, statements regarding copyright credits appear in the appropriate places in the text.

The material on behavior therapy in Chapters 12 through 15 represents an expanded version of a chapter I contributed to the *Manual of Child Psychopathology*, edited by Benjamin B. Wolman and published by McGraw-Hill in 1972. Doctor Wolman and our mutual publisher kindly agreed to my basing the "treatment" chapters on this work, and I appreciate that they thus made it unnecessary for me to paraphrase my own writing.

Alan O. Ross

PSYCHOLOGICAL DISORDERS OF CHILDREN

PART I

PRINCIPLES OF PSYCHOLOGICAL DISORDERS

1

INTRODUCTION

THE BEHAVIORAL APPROACH

In *Essay on Man* Alexander Pope exclaimed, "The proper study of mankind is man." To this the psychologist might add, "The proper study of man is man's behavior." When a scientist desires to study a natural phenomenon, this phenomenon must be observable. Speculation may serve him for a while, but ultimately these speculations must be confirmed through observation. Similarly, indirect observation of a phenomenon may, for a time, be all the scientist has available, but ultimately direct observation will be necessary if his inferences are to be confirmed. In the case of the natural phenomenon that is the human being, the only thing we can observe is his behavior. Man's history is the record of man's behavior. When man constructs tools, builds houses, creates works of art, speaks to other men, or teaches his children, man is emitting behavior. Behavior can be observed and recorded, hence, scientifically studied, and this scientific study of behavior is psychology, the science of behavior.

All behavior, whether sublime or profane, unique or commonplace, normal or deviant, follows the same principles. Many of these principles are now known while others remain to be discovered; yet, enough of them are known to venture a presentation of the psychological disorders of children based on the behavior principles of psychology. The aim of this presentation is to arrive at an explanation of these disorders through the application of behavior principles, an explanation which will hopefully contribute to alleviating the disorders and preventing them from developing.

Explanation and Understanding

The observation of a puzzling phenomenon, such as a child who repeatedly bangs his head against the wall to the point where he sustains large swellings and lacerated skin, leads layman and psychologist alike to seek an explanation. The kind of explanation one finds greatly depends on the kind of question one asks. If the question is "What makes a child behave like this?", the answer is likely to be in terms of something that *makes* the child bang his head, something that impels, motivates, or forces him to act this way. What is more, the search for an answer is likely to focus on antecedent events, on looking for an entity that is present inside the child and pushes him to do what he does. Over the years a variety of such causes have been invented to explain the puzzling behavior. These have ranged from inherent evil, through malevolent spirits, to inherited wickedness and unconscious conflicts. Each of these explanatory fictions has, in its time, served to give people the sense of understanding puzzling behavior, but the science of psychology cannot be satisfied with pseudoexplanations which do not lend themselves to experimental manipulations and have no referent, independent of the phenomenon they seek to explain. What is more, these pseudoexplanations have done little in way of helping the children whose behavior they purport to explain, and such help is the most important reason for seeking an explanation. From that standpoint, more recent explanations in terms of such constructs as personality and character traits have also done little to improve the approaches used to modify changeworthy behavior.

If the "what" question leads one to invent homunculi and mysterious forces, the "why" question ("Why does the child bang his head?") is likely to produce equally fallacious answers. The focus is now shifted from an impelling force to an attracting goal; the child bangs his head in order to satisfy some need, urge, or impulse. To solve the "why" question, this need must then be identified, and people have again turned to inventions for an answer. One of the most frequently encountered pseudoexplanations here is the explanatory label. The observed behavior is given a label—the more esoteric, the better; and this label then comes to serve as an explanation. In the case of the head-banging child, the behavior might be called *masochistic*, and the question "Why does the child bang his head?" then receives the answer "Because he is masochistic" or "Because it satisfies his masochistic needs." When this explanation is challenged ("How do you know he has masochistic needs?") the answer returns to the observation which was to be explained in the first place ("Because he bangs his head"). The circularity of this should be obvious, but many of the explanatory constructs still in use in psychology are of that order.

Aside from encouraging the postulation of needs that have no external referent other than the phenomenon to be explained, the "why" question is also likely to trap one into teleological explanations. These explanations infer a purpose, an intention, or a plan that antedates the emission of the behavior; the child bangs his head "in order to" gain some satisfying goal that he was able to envision beforehand. A behavioral approach to psychology does not deny that people make plans and engage in behavior that follows such a plan. The problem is that the presence or absence of such a plan cannot be directly studied, and it is risky to infer the presence of a plan from observed behavior because topographically similar behavior may appear in the presence as well as in the absence of a plan. A nonverbal, severely disturbed child who bangs his head is not likely to tell us the purpose of his behavior, and to postulate such a purpose is not the most parsimonious route to a satisfactory explanation.

To summarize what has been said so far, an analogy might be helpful. If one observes that the sun appears in the sky in the morning and asks, "What makes the sun rise?", the answer might be, "The sun-god Helios is driving his 4-horse chariot through the heavens." If one were to rephrase the question and ask, "Why does the sun rise?", the answer might be, "In order to make daylight." Neither the "what" nor the "why" question is appropriate for science. The only causal question science can investigate takes the form, "Under what conditions does this phenomenon occur?"

Returning to the head-banging child, we can now ask, "Under what conditions does this child bang his head?", and the psychologist can proceed to observe the phenomenon in question and to gather data on the events immediately preceding and immediately following the behavior. This will lead him to discover that the behavior is a function of environmental conditions and that, when he modifies these conditions, he can modify the behavior. When the full answer to the question about the conditions surrounding a given behavior is available, the behavior can be predicted and, under given circumstances, controlled—that is, created, changed, or prevented. These are the goals of science—prediction and control. When these goals are reached, one can say that an observed phenomenon is explained or, if one likes, "understood." Understanding in any other sense is scientifically meaningless although philosophers, theologians, and artists—in laudable pursuits of their endeavors—will and should seek an understanding of the world in other terms. A discussion of behavior disorders must seek a scientific understanding because such understanding alone permits us to modify and, ultimately, to prevent problems of this nature.

Determinants of Behavior

The question about the conditions under which a given phenomenon takes place leads the behavioral psychologist to study the external environment. This is not to deny that there are also conditions of the internal environment which deserve study, and the biologically oriented psychologist, the physiologist, and the biochemist can study these to great advantage. It is fallacious to assume, however, that an "ultimate" explanation of behavior can be found on the molecular, physiological level. Any specific behavior, taking place at any one point, represents the end point of the interaction of genetic-constitutional factors, the current physiological state of the individual, his current environmental conditions and past learning which, in turn, was a function of a similar interaction. All four of these inter-acting factors must be explored; to assume that any one alone will provide a necessary and sufficient explanation is to ignore the com-plexity of the phenomenon that is human behavior.

Genetic-Constitutional Factors Each individual possesses unique attributes of a biological order. Some of these attributes he has in common with other members of the species, and they probably evolved and became a part of the human behavioral repertoire because of their survival value. Simple reflexes, the avoidance of noxious stimulation, and the escape from danger are examples of genotypical behavior that is largely a function of innate, genetic endowment. Other attributes, such as his pain threshold, his au-tonomic reactivity, and his behavioral style, seem to be aspects of the individual's phenotypical uniqueness. An individual's attributes are probably present at the time of birth and may be viewed as hereditary in the sense that they represent the interplay of his parents' genes. With the exception of identical twins, every individual differs from every other individual in terms of the exact combination of genetic attributes, and any study of behavior must take these individual differences into consideration. While the science of ge-netics has made much progress in recent years, we do not, at this point in time, have enough knowledge to permit a clear differentia-tion between genotypical and phenotypical factors, and this lack of knowledge leads us to refer to those behavioral aspects with which a child appears to be born as *constitutional.* At this point, too, we are unable to influence these constitutional factors before they emerge, although, within limits, they can later be modified and brought under voluntary control. Thus, an individual can learn to make approach responses in the face of danger or noxious stimuli, to increase his pain tolerance, or to modify such autonomic responses as heart rate or blood pressure (Katkin & Murray, 1968).

Past Learning Another factor influencing present behavior is the person's past learning with respect to similar situations. All behavior, with the possible exception of the simple reflex, is either developed by or modified through learning. When we observe a specific response, we see the end result of a long history of learning. A person will behave in a given situation largely in terms of his past learning in similar situations, and his behavior will be predictable to the extent that this past learning and its conditions can be known. In real life it is next to impossible to reconstruct the conditions under which a person has learned and to know the nature of this learning; hence, human behavior is difficult to predict, but the best predictor is knowledge of past behavior under similar circumstances. This is the case because behavior depends on the prevailing environmental conditions and is specific to these conditions. People do not carry response dispositions around with them from place to place, and thus they do not respond in the same manner, no matter what the place. Attempts to assess response dispositions (character traits or personality states) in hopes of facilitating the prediction of behavior have been singularly unsuccessful (Mischel, 1968). By definition, past learning is *past* and thus not subject to cancellation; that is, it cannot be made to have not happened. It potently influences present behavior, yet we cannot hope to change present behavior by merely exploring past learning. We can, however, modify the effects of past learning by introducing new learning, thereby modifying future behavior under similar circumstances.

Current Physiological State   At the moment an individual emits a specific behavior, he is in a physiological state that plays a role in the behavior. Physiological states may be constitutional and thus of relative permanence, as blood pressure, for example, or they may be such temporary states as level of food deprivation or degree of autonomic arousal. These physiological factors affect the person's behavior. For example, for a person who is not to some extent deprived of food, the opportunity to eat is not a reinforcing state of affairs; a person who is not at least mildly aroused may not respond to the presentation of a given signal that, at other times, would serve him as a stimulus. While physiological factors are thus preconditions or setting events for behavior, they themselves have their antecedents in environmental circumstances. Food deprivation (hunger) is a function of something going on in the environment, and arousal states are responses to a variety of stimuli such as sleep deprivation, threat, or stress. Since the environmental antecedents of an individual's physiological state are thus subject to modification, it is possible to modify the physiological state if one desires to modify the individual's behavior.

Current Environmental Conditions The fourth interacting influence on current behavior, and of greatest interest to the behaviorally oriented psychologist, is the condition under which current behavior takes place. The immediate antecedents and the immediate consequences of a given action are present in the here and now; they can be observed, recorded, measured, counted, and otherwise made the subject matter of the science of behavior. What is more, current environmental conditions, unlike genetic factors or past learning, can be modified to influence not only behavior but also the physiological states that affect behavior.

The focus on behavior and the environment in which the behavior takes place lends itself not only to providing an understanding of behavior and behavior disorders, it also furnishes guidelines to those who seek to modify behavior disorders in a therapeutic endeavor. A study of behavior disorders that does not logically lead to their treatment would be no more than abstract theorizing, and there is too much human suffering involved to permit one the luxury of such esoteric pursuits.

The main principles we shall invoke in discussing the acquisition and change of behavior are the principles of respondent conditioning and vicarious and operant learning. These will be briefly reviewed at the beginning of the section dealing with the treatment of psychological disorders (Chapter 12), for it is there that their pragmatic implications can be immediately recognized. It is, however, important to keep in mind that while these principles of learning have been shown to work when they are applied in the *modification* of disordered behavior, this is no proof that these principles are necessarily involved in the *development* of such behavior. The assumption is that disordered behavior is a function of learning and that principles of learning operate there as they do in treatment, but support for this assumption cannot be adduced by pointing to the data from behavior modification. We shall repeatedly warn against the fallacy of *post hoc, ergo propter hoc*.

Because of obvious ethical constraints one cannot produce behavior disorders for the purpose of demonstrating how they develop; laboratory analogues occasionally lend some support, but, ultimately, only painstaking longitudinal studies tracing the development of behavior disorders and recording all contributing conditions will permit us to be confident about statements on the genesis of psychological disorders.

Private Events

In the behavioral approach to psychological phenomena, one prefers to study that which can be observed or made observable. Overt behavior—what people do, what they say, and how they look—thus provides the primary data; in addition, such physiological events as changes in heart rate, skin conductance, or respiration which can be objectively recorded provide information about functions which are not visible to the observer without the aid of specialized equipment. Observed overt behavior as well as recorded physiological events can be described in objective terms; they can be seen by any number of observers who can agree on what they are seeing, and they can be communicated to others who can repeat the observations, given similar circumstances. Objectivity, communicability, and repeatability are the requisites of a science, and the data gathered by a behavioral approach thus permit the development of scientific knowledge about psychological phenomena. As information thus obtained accumulates, one can discover that certain discrete behavioral events coincide with great predictability with certain discrete physiological events, and at this point communication among investigators can be facilitated if, instead of continuing to list the discrete observations, they agree on a linguistic convention whereby this cluster of events is given a label. One can observe, for example, that many people when prevented from the completion of a goal-oriented response chain will increase the magnitude of certain motor responses; show a characteristic facial grimace; emit verbal expletives and statements like "I am angry"; develop a flushing of the facial skin; and have concomitant changes in heart rate, blood pressure, skin conductance, or breathing pattern, which can be displayed on specialized equipment. This cluster of observed phenomena can be called "anger," and such a term can then be used in discussions of behavior, provided one recalls that it stands not for a postulated internal state but for a series of observable phenomena and that it is these observations (operations) which define the term. Such operational definitions can be worked out for anxiety, joy, sadness, hunger, and other internal responses, but unless these have observable referents, the terms alone have no scientific standing.

Terms like anger, sadness, or hunger are a part of the general English vocabulary, and this creates some confusion because people describe their own sensations in these terms thereby giving the impression that, when used in the technical language of psychology, they also refer directly to internal states and are not merely convenient semantic conventions describing a defined set of observations. This confusion might have been avoided had psychologists decided to designate observed clusters of behavior by some arcane term especially invented for the purpose, but this would have prevented one confusion by creating another. At any rate, when a person tells us that he is angry, he tells us something about a private experience. But to the psychologist this verbal statement is merely one of many defining characteristics of the behavior cluster he has agreed to call anger, and unless the remaining characteristics can also be demonstrated, the psychologist in his role as scientist must guard against accepting the verbal statement alone as a reliable index of the presence of the behavior cluster. This caveat is particularly important when we come to discuss the behavior of children because young or severely disturbed children may not have words to describe their sensations or may be using such words in highly idiosyncratic ways.

The words with which we describe perceived internal states are learned in the course of language acquisition. Children learn the verbal labels for concrete external referents with relative ease. The object called "horse" can be pointed to by a parent who says "horse," and when the child eventually repeats this word, he can be rewarded or, if on occasion, he calls it "cow," he can be corrected. It is far more difficult to teach verbal labels for internal events because parent and child do not have a common referent, and the parent is unable to provide the child with feedback as to the accuracy of his statement. For this reason the language dealing with subjective states is far more unreliable than the language about the objective world. Some people describe as anger what others might label anxiety; others say they are embarrassed when someone else might report feeling guilty, and, as we have said, children very often have no words at all to describe their internal sensations. Thus, while an inquiry into how a person "feels" may be useful in eliciting one of the observable behaviors (the verbal statement), by itself the answer is of little value in the study of disordered behavior.

The behaviorally oriented psychologist does not deny that people experience internal sensations; he merely considers the verbal reports of such sensations highly suspect data, and he refuses to make inferences about internal states, preferring instead to deal with what he can observe. The same is true about the private events called *thoughts, fantasies, ideas, wishes, plans, memories,* etc. There is no doubt that people engage in these cognitive processes, but the only way in which a psychologist can study them is by observing behavior (including verbal behavior) that accompanies these processes. Again, it is necessary to have more than a verbal self-report before a private event can furnish useful data. Self-reports may be inaccurate, withheld, distorted, or falsified, and the non-verbal or preverbal child has no way of giving such a report. From the point of view of psychology it is more useful to record the observation that a child flaps his arms, makes chirping noises, and so doing jumps off high places than to have him tell us that he thinks he is a bird; but if all of these events are observed, it may help communication to make the statement that this child has bird fantasies. A therapist would undoubtedly wish to change the child's deviant and dangerous behavior regardless of the nature of the fantasy; and, as we shall see, it is possible to bring about such change without inquiring into or making inferences about the fantasies which may or may not be present and about which we can have no direct knowledge unless the child is willing and able to give us a verbal statement with reference to them.

To summarize, the behaviorally oriented psychologist does not deny the existence of such private events as thoughts and feelings; he merely maintains that self-reports about such private events provide unreliable data, insists that their reliability must be enhanced by concurrently observed behavior before they can be used in a scientific study of psychological phenomena, and prefers, as a matter of strategy, to focus his attention on what he can observe or make observable.

PSYCHOLOGICAL DISORDERS
There is no absolute definition of a psychological disorder. The definition is a function of the social environment and thus relative to the cultural, historical, and social setting in which an individual emits a given behavior. If the behavior conforms to the prevailing con-sensual norm, it is considered *normal*; if it deviates from this norm, it is considered *deviant*. In a given society, at any given time in its history, the members of that society have fairly explicit expectations for the role-appropriate behavior of a child. These expectations are a function of the child's age, and they vary depending on his sex, position in birth order, and the social status of his family. The child whose behavior deviates from these expectations, whose behavior does not fit into the expected order of the lives of those with whom he lives, and whose behavior is thus "disordered" finds himself exposed to sanctions imposed by his peers and elders. These sanctions will be brought to bear if the behavior is emitted under conditions where it is deemed "improper" (literally, "where it does not belong"), for a given action may be appropriate in one set of circumstances but inappropriate in another. What is more, a behavior may be deemed acceptable when it is performed at one level of frequency or magnitude but unacceptable at higher or lower levels. Thus, for example, a parent may approve of his child's hitting another child only if he has been hit first and only if the other child is at least his age. Furthermore, occasional hitting of another on the part of a nine-year-old boy is usually tolerated, but when this occurs very

often, it is deemed a problem, particularly if his family is of middle-class status.

With these points in mind, it is possible to propose the following *definition of psychological disorders:*

> A psychological disorder is said to be present when a child emits behavior that deviates from a discretionary and relative social norm in that it occurs with a frequency or intensity that authoritative adults in the child's environment judge, under the circumstances, to be either too high or too low.

Peers, parents, and other adults in the child's environment will impose sanctions for deviant behavior; they withhold positive reinforcement or deliver noxious stimuli. Yet in the face of these negative consequences, the disordered behavior persists in the child's repertoire, giving such behavior its characteristic maladaptive, paradoxical nature. Despite repeated failure, frequent punishment, loss of friends, and absence of apparent rewards, the child persists to engage in the acts which have these consequences, and this paradox leads most observers to wonder what it is that "makes" the child behave in this manner. They seek to understand and explain the paradox, and this search leads, as we have seen, to a variety of formulations.

At present, the most parsimonious approach to an understanding of disordered behavior is to view such behavior as acquired, performed, and modifiable according to the same principles of development and learning that apply to all other behavior. From this standpoint, one can attempt to resolve the paradox of maladaptive behavior by assuming that such behavior is maintained by indirect or delayed forms of reinforcement that are not mysterious but just not immediately apparent to the casual observer. The task of psychology then becomes to identify these reinforcing conditions, for by changing these conditions one should be able to modify the disordered behavior. In addition to disordered behavior that is probably maintained by indirect or delayed reinforcement, there is a group of behavior disorders where the child has never learned appropriate, expected response patterns in the course of his development. He, too, will encounter negative consequences of his behavior so that it may appear paradoxical, but because punishment can, at best, serve to suppress behavior and cannot teach new, appropriate responses, his persistence in the maladaptive pattern is not a mystery but a reflection of his deficient response repertoire. Here, the task of psychology is to find ways of teaching the child the skills he has so far failed to acquire.

The behavior which our present society chooses to define as disordered falls into two major classes, depending on whether, in the eyes of those who judge the child, he emits too little or too much of a particular behavior. One can thus speak of *deficient behavior* and *excess behavior*, and this dichotomy will be used in our presentation of behavior disorders. Within these classes a variety of categories can be distinguished. Thus, excess behavior can take two forms: it can involve excessive approach responses or excessive avoidance responses. The former, when emitted at high magnitude, we can call aggressive behavior, the latter, withdrawn behavior. Deficient behavior is marked by its inadequacy in the face of social and environmental demands. At the present time, our society is particularly sensitive to inadequacy in the areas of intelligence and self-control, and problems in these areas are highlighted by special labels. When the child is inadequate in the area of intelligence, we speak of mental subnormality; when difficulty in self-control reaches intolerable proportions, we recognize the norm-violating behavior of the juvenile delinquent. These and other labels will serve as chapter headings for our discussion, but, as will be apparent, they are not entities but merely convenient summary terms for behavior clusters. Some of these behavior clusters reflect statistically definable patterns, and the following chapter will be devoted to a review of studies by which investigators have attempted to establish such patterns in hopes of classifying psychological disorders of children.

2

THE CLASSIFICATION OF PSYCHOLOGICAL DISORDERS

Attempts to establish a taxonomy of psychological disorders would be an idle intellectual exercise were it not for the fact that there are several pragmatic questions, the answers to which await the development of a uniform system of classification. In order to study what kind of treatment works best with what kind of disorder, one must be able to define "kinds of disorders." If two investigators wish to compare data, they must be able to agree on the disorders they are discussing. If one wishes to ascertain the incidence of a particular disorder in a given population, one must have a taxonomic basis for conducting the survey. Lastly, if one desires to write a textbook on the psychological disorders of children, one needs a systematic way of ordering the available information.

All of these efforts are presently handicapped by the lack of a uniformly agreed upon system of classifying the psychological disorders of children. There are many reasons for this state of affairs, some of which will become apparent from the following pages; but the prime reason why we are still in the pre-Linnaean stage of our science is that there has been all manner of confusion about the nature of the phenomenon we wish to classify. Is a psychological disorder a disease, in which case one would want to follow the medical approach to classification and nomenclature? Are childrens' disorders analogous to adults' disorders, in which case the reasonably uniform nomenclature used there might be applied with only minor modifications? Should one base the classification on the manifestations of the problem, on its origins, on its effect on others, or on its probable outcome? Each of these possibilities and combinations of them have, at one time or other, served as the basis of attempts at classification but none have proved satisfactory.

The phenomenon we wish to classify is, of course, not an object or an entity; it is the behavior and combinations of behaviors emitted by individual children whose social environment judges the behavior to be deviant. Attempts to reify behavior or to deal with it by analogy would seem to be the main reason why the classification of behavior disorders—and with it, the study of such disorders—has failed to progress.

A system for classifying psychological disorders must be based on "meaningful and discernible behaviors" (Zigler & Phillips, 1961). The classificatory principle must be consistently organized around observable behavior; references to etiology, prognosis, social conformity, developmental stage, etc., must be explicitly stated as correlates of the particular behavior or class of behaviors. Zigler and Phillips (1961) in their critique of psychiatric diagnosis pointed out that present classificatory systems tend to confound diverse principles of classification. A formulation advanced by the Committee on Child Psychiatry of the Group for the Advancement of Psychiatry (1966) is a case in point, for it attempts a classification that mixes principles of behavior (reactive disorders), age (developmental deviations), severity (psychotic disorders), and etiology (brain syndromes).

When a psychological disorder is defined in terms of a judgment made by the child's environment, such judgments become central to any system of classification. In fact, one might say that we must classify not behavior but people's judgments about behavior. For when it is recognized that the definition of disordered behavior depends on the expectations of a child's environment, it becomes clear that one must consider not only the demands this environment makes of the child but also the tolerance level of this environment for behavior in its various forms. The data for classifying psychological disorders of children should therefore be the reports of those who, like parents and teachers, are in daily contact with the child. This leads us to a consideration of what, in child behavior, parents and teachers will judge to be disordered, and what they judge to be normal behavior of children.

WHAT IS NORMAL?

As a first approximation of a differentiation between disordered and normal behavior, one might assume that behavior which causes a child to be brought to the attention of a relevant professional is abnormal, while the behavior of children in the nonclinic population is normal. It should be immediately apparent that this is a poor basis on which to make the differentiation. The arbitrary and relative nature of what people consider to be a behavior disorder should lead one to suspect that the same behavior can be found on either side of the clinic door.

The children who come to professional attention represent a highly selected, biased sample of those who manifest a given behavior, and any studies based on these children must be viewed with this fact clearly in mind. The prevalence of the kind of behavior which brings children to the attention of relevant clinics and agencies has been shown to be remarkably high in unselected samples of the so-called normal population (Conners, 1970; Lapouse & Monk, 1959, 1964; Werry & Quay, 1971).

In a survey of all children attending kindergarten through second grade in the public schools of a town in Illinois, Werry and Quay (1971) used a 55-item checklist containing problems found among children brought to child guidance clinics. These ranged from shyness to disruptiveness, from temper tantrums to bizarre behavior. The children's teachers were asked to check those behaviors they recognized in a given child, and the authors report that the mean number of such problems was 11.4 for the 926 boys and 7.6 for the 827 girls in the sample. The significantly higher incidence of problems among boys is a finding reported with great consistency by most investigators. In the Illinois study, thirty-six of the problems occurred with significantly greater frequency among boys; only five problems were more frequent among girls. These were shyness, seriousness, jealousy, sensitivity, and physical complaints.

Conners (1970) conducted a comparison of 316 children who were attending a psychiatric clinic and 365 presumably normal children whose parents were attending a PTA meeting. He used a list of seventy-three problem behaviors on which the parents of the children checked the problems displayed by their child. While, as expected, the prevalence of problems was higher among the clinic patients than among the normal sample, some difficulties had a surprisingly high prevalence among the so-called normal children. Thus, their parents checked "restlessness" for 65 percent of the children; bed-wetting for 15 percent; nightmares for 24 percent; overeating for 11 percent; and biting, sucking, or chewing objects for 20 percent. While parents who attend PTA meetings represent a select sample of the general population of parents and may be somewhat more interested in and concerned about their child's welfare, Conners' data are remarkably consistent with those reported by Lapouse and Monk (1959). They found that in a sample of 482 children between the ages of six and twelve—carefully selected to represent the general population of a city in New York State—17 percent wet their bed, 28 percent had nightmares, 27 percent bit their nails, and 43 percent experienced seven or more fears and worries out of thirty about which their mothers had been questioned.

The Louisville Behavior Check List (Miller, 1967a, 1967b) contains 163 statements describing both deviant and prosocial behavior in nontechnical language. When parents or teachers are asked to check the items which are descriptive of a given child, this instrument yields scores on eight scales in the areas of aggression, withdrawal, and learning disabilities as well as an overall "total disability" score which is based on ninety-three items that have been found to contribute to the other eight scales. This checklist and its predecessor, the Pittsburgh Adjustment Survey Scales (Ross, Lacey, & Parton, 1965), have been found to be reliable and to have a stable factor structure. Miller, Hampe, Barrett, and

Noble (1971) mailed the Louisville Behavior Check List to a random sample of 500 parents of children between the ages of seven and twelve, drawn from the rolls of the city and county public school systems in and around Louisville. With mail and telephone follow-up they secured a 47 percent return, yielding 236 protocols. The analysis of the responses from this random sample of the general population revealed that "the average child within the general population manifests between 11 and 13 deviant behaviors" (p. 18), deviant behavior items occurring in at least 25 percent of the population. The scales were only minimally affected by such demographic variables as race, socioeconomic status, and age, and there were no significant differences between the total disability means for boys and girls, although the scores for boys had a higher variance. That is to say that boys manifested more extreme behavior than girls, particularly on the aggressive and learning disability dimensions. The scales reflecting academic disability and immaturity, scales Miller and his associates classify as learning disability, did show significantly higher means for boys than for girls. This finding, together with the negative correlation between intelligence and disability scores, led the authors to speculate that much disturbed behavior in childhood "may be linked to scholastic failures resulting from an incompatibility between children of lower intelligence and the modern educational system" (p. 21).

The most significant finding of the Louisville study would seem to be that scores for boys and girls were similar except in the area of learning disorders. Miller et al. (1971) point out that this stands in sharp contrast to the sex ratios among children referred to clinics which, in study after study, has shown an excess of boys over girls of the order of 3 to 1. Similarly, both informal reports and systematic studies (Peterson, 1961; Werry & Quay, 1971) have shown that teachers have more trouble with boys than with girls. A possible explanation for this discrepancy, offered by Miller et al., is in line with the thinking underlying this chapter: It is the tolerance of significant adults in the child's environment and not some absolute standard of normality that provides the basis for a definition of behavior disorders. Recalling that the boys in their sample were more extreme in their behavior and that they also had greater difficulty with formal learning, the authors suggest that the basic problem is in failure to learn. When failure occurs in boys, their reaction is more likely to find expression in aggression, hyperactivity, and antisocial behavior. When failure occurs in girls, their reaction is more likely to be manifested in social withdrawal, sensitivity, and fear. "Since children are often referred when they become problems to adults, and since aggression is more likely to become a problem to adults, boys are more likely to be referred for treatment" (p. 21). The fact that a high incidence of learning disorders is found in treatment clinics which also have a high male/female ratio would seem to lend support to this speculation. The strong interaction between learning disorders and problem behaviors may also explain the discrepancy between the results reported by Werry and Quay (1971) and those of Miller and his associates. Werry and Quay, it will be recalled, used teachers as respondents and found a higher incidence of problems among boys while the latter, having gathered their data from checklists filled out by parents, failed to find such a difference. Assuming that the responses of parents and of teachers are equally valid, it may be that compared to girls, boys, who have more difficulty with learning, find school a more aversive situation and respond to that situation with behaviors viewed by their teachers as aggressive, hyperactive, or antisocial. Since behavior is largely situation-specific and not carried from situation to situation in the form of a "trait," these same boys may behave differently under the stimulus conditions prevalent in their homes where their parents would rate their behavior as being no more problematic than that of girls.

The normative information provided by their random sample of the general population together with data from an earlier study based on a clinic population, permitted Miller, Hampe, Barrett, and Noble (1971) to set statistical cutoff scores at one and two standard deviations above the mean, respectively. A disability score of 25 (1σ above the mean) classified 85 percent of the general population as nondisturbed, while a disability score of 37 (2σ above the mean) accounted for 98 percent of the general population. This, in turn, permits an estimate of the number of children in the total child population who might be expected to obtain scores in the disturbed range. Assuming that there are 26 million children in the United States between the ages of six and twelve, Miller et al. make the projection that there are one-half million children with a disability score of 25 in this age group. Put in another way, 15 out of every 100 parents in the community will attribute a disability score of at least 25 to their children. Since the best available estimate places at 1,800 the number of professional child mental health workers in the United States, this would mean a professional/child ratio of 1 to 8,000 for these children. Miller and his colleagues rightly state that "these numbers stagger the imagination" (1971, p. 22).

The high prevalence in the normal population of behaviors that are viewed as problems for children brought for professional help raises the question of what happens to these behaviors when they are not defined as problems calling for intervention. At present the answer to that is not known. To get it one would have to survey an unselected population of children, using someone other than a parent as respondent, and then repeat this survey on the same children at intervals over a number of years. Such a study has not been done so that the question of what becomes of a given behavior which does not interfere with a child's adaptation or which no one in his environment considers a problem remains unanswered.

Once a behavior is designated as a problem, there is some indication (Levitt, 1957, 1963) that approximately two-thirds of the children with such problems improve within 2 years without professional intervention. It seems that as a child and his environment undergo changes, so that the reinforcement contingencies for his behavior change, problematic behavior tends to drop out of the repertoire. If this is true of problems which are identified as such, one can assume that it is also true of behaviors that have not been viewed as problems.

The issue of normality and its converse, the question of when a behavior is a problem, has a number of other ramifications (Ross, 1963), not the least of which is the validity of the judgment made by the people in the child's environment about any particular aspect of his behavior. One must be concerned not only with the question "When is a behavior a problem?" but also with "When is a problem not a child's behavior disorder?" When the tolerance level of a child's environment is an important factor in the definition of a behavior disorder, then this tolerance level can also be too high or too low. If it is too low, parents may seek help around a behavior of their child that few others in their community would deem problematic, and the professional person to whom they come for help must thus exercise a judgment that will involve his norms, standards, and values. There are times when the parents' tolerance level and not the child's behavior is to be changed. One must also remember that some behaviors which a child's adult environment deems problematic is, in fact, an adaptive response to a problematic environment. Thus, in the survey by Werry and Quay (1971), half of the boys (49.7 percent) in the presumably normal kindergarten, first, and second grade classes in the public school system were reported as displaying "restlessness, inability to sit still"; "distractibility" was checked for 48.2 percent of the boys; and 46.3 percent of the boys were charged with "disruptiveness, tendency to annoy others." It makes little sense to speak of behavior problems when nearly half of an unselected population engages in that form of behavior. If one uses the statistical concept of normality, the restless, distractible, and disruptive behavior of the children in this school system would have to be viewed as normal behavior. But the teachers check it off on a problem ("symptom") checklist. Whose problem is it? Could it be that classrooms in elementary school are so structured and teacher behavior so programmed that the "normal," to be expected behavior of male children is to emit responses the teacher identifies as restlessness and distractibility? If this is the case, the modification called for is situational-environmental and should not have its focus on changing the behavior of the boys so that they "adjust" to what may be an intolerable situation.

With the arbitrary and relative nature of the definition of psychological disorders clearly in mind, we turn now to a review of studies which represent attempts to contribute to a taxonomy of behavior disorders, using descriptions of behavior as basic data.

TOWARD A TAXONOMY OF BEHAVIOR DISORDERS

A number of investigators have taken the observations of parents or teachers as the basis for classifying psychological disorders of children. These observations can be recorded as responses on behavior checklists, or they can be the complaints around which children are presented to clinics specializing in work with psychological disorders. While none of the studies to be reviewed has led to a comprehensive system of classification, the results of studies of this nature may contribute to the eventual development of such a system.

Factor Analysis

The observations or complaints that parents and teachers report regarding the behavior of children can take a great many forms, and the words that might be used, including synonyms and euphemisms, probably number in the thousands. It is therefore necessary to reduce these descriptive statements to manageable size and to attempt to order them along some logical dimension. The statistical method of factor analysis permits the ordering of large numbers of discrete observations by identifying the nature of their interrelationship.

There are, for example, 163 statements in the Louisville Behavior Check List (Miller, 1967b), each describing a specific behavior that a child might be observed to emit. When parents are asked to indicate on this checklist which behaviors are descriptive of their child, they might pick as many as forty, some identifying deviant, some prosocial, behavior. When an investigator has collected many such checklists from a large sample of parents, he will find that certain items on his list tend to be checked together; that is, they tend to correlate. For instance, on a checklist developed by Ross, Lacey, and Parton (1965), such items as "He teases other children," "He hits and pushes other children," and "He boasts about how tough he is" were usually checked together—when one item applied to a given child, the others would usually also apply. On the other hand, such items as "He becomes frightened easily," "He is afraid of making mistakes," and "He is easily upset by changes in things around him" were rarely checked with the earlier items but were, in turn, often checked together with each other and similar items.

A factor analysis identifies such intercorrelated clusters of items (factors), and the investigator can then give these factors a descriptive label and derive scales that make up his instrument. In the example given above, the first set of items belongs to the aggressive-behavior scale, the second set to the withdrawn-behavior scale of the checklist.

In an attempt to derive a classificatory system by means of a factor analysis, the investigator must make a number of decisions at various stages of his study. Some of these decisions will have critical effects on the results. The question of what statements to include in the basic instrument is solved differently by different investigators. Some use statements derived from the complaints with which parents bring their children to the attention of clinicians; others collect observations of child behavior and then prepare descriptive statements on the basis of these observations. Some use statements which require that the respondent make a subjective judgment, while others attempt to write statements that require no inferences on the part of the person filling out the questionnaire. Again, some investigators include only problem behaviors, while others purposely write items describing nonproblematic, so-called prosocial behavior. Some choose to omit items referring to academic performance, thereby hoping to avoid a negative halo effect whereby the poor student would also be viewed as emitting problem behaviors, while others purposely include such items, wishing to identify learning difficulties together with other behavior problems.

After an investigator has answered the question of what items to include in his instrument, he has to make other crucial decisions, such as what population to study, how to compose his sample, and whom to use as respondents. After the data are gathered, certain technical decisions arise, such as which of several factor-analytic methods to use and how many factors to extract. Finally, after component factors have been identified, the investigator must decide whether to give these factors descriptive labels and, if so, what to call them.

Among the decisions of research strategy that will influence the results of a factor analytic study is the choice of subject population. If one surveys the behavior of children who are referred to a child guidance clinic, maladaptive behavior will be found with a high frequency, but the number of children available for such study will be limited by the relatively small case load of such a clinic. Some investigators (e.g., Hewitt & Jenkins, 1946) have attempted to increase the number of children available for study by surveying the case histories in clinic files, but this approach suffers from the weakness found in any research using data not originally gathered for research purposes. Peterson (1961) decided to obtain the large number of subjects necessary for meaningful statistical analysis by sampling from the unselected public school population. While this approach resulted in 957 ratings, it brought with it the problem of low frequency of the more profound behavior disorders which occur rarely among children attending public school but are frequently found in clinic populations. It was therefore necessary to exclude such problems as soiling and enuresis, and to consider as of equal weight problems rated mild and problems rated severe. It has been suggested (Ross, 1959) that the best way of assuring an adequate number of subjects for research on clinical problems would be the pooling of cases from two or more collaborating clinics. This approach was used by Dreger et al. (1964) who succeeded in having thirteen child guidance clinics systematically gather data in a uniform manner for the Behavioral Classification Project. This ambitious project unfortunately suffered weaknesses (discussed below) that make its results difficult to evaluate.

Yet another strategy decision affecting the outcome of factor analytic studies of behavior problems is the choice of items to be intercorrelated. Validity is enhanced if the items to be rated or counted describe specific behaviors on the presence or absence of which two or more observers can readily agree. The more concrete and specific an individual item, however, the longer will have to be the list of items, and the greater the likelihood of very low or zero frequencies which will skew the distribution of ratings. Such high specificity of items appears to have been one of the difficulties in the Behavioral Classification Project directed by Dreger (1964), whose list contained 229 strictly behavioral items requiring no inference or abstraction on the part of the respondent. Peterson (1961), on the other hand, chose to base his list of fifty-eight items on common referral problems including such abstractions as "feelings of inferiority." Achenbach (1966) strove for a compromise between specificity and abstraction by using items requiring as little inference as possible without being excessively molecular. This led to a list of ninety-one referral problems for which he searched clinic records in order to obtain data for the factor analytic study which will be discussed below.

The Direction of Behavior

Because investigators differ in the decisions they make at these various choice-points, their studies are difficult to compare and their results are sometimes contradictory. Despite this, two general categories of excess maladaptive behavior appear with an impressive frequency in diverse empirical studies (Achenbach, 1966; Conners, 1970; Dreger et al., 1964; Miller, 1968; Patterson, 1964; Peterson, 1961; Ross et al., 1965) as well as in deductive discussions (Ackerson, 1931; Ross, 1959). These categories differentiate excess approach behavior (aggression) and excess avoidance behavior (withdrawal). Different investigators give different labels to these categories, but they invariably revolve around the direction of the maladaptive responses, toward or away from the environment. The terms used to describe this dichotomy often reflect the writer's theoretical orientation. Kessler (1966) speaks of the effect of the disturbance and asks, "Who suffers?", the child or other people; Peterson (1961) writes, "In one case, impulses are expressed and society suffers; in the other case impulses are evidently inhibited and the child suffers" (p. 206) and speaks of these two classes as "conduct problems" and "personality problems." Achenbach (1966) labeled his bipolar factor internalizing versus externalizing so as to describe "conflict with the environment" as against "problems within the self" (p. 10). Studies that resulted in a more complex factor structure (Patterson, 1964; Dreger et al., 1964) include behavior clusters that can be recognized as subsuming children whose maladaptive behavior is expressed toward the environment (aggression) and those who retreat from social interaction (withdrawal). Scales developed to measure these two dimensions (Ross, Lacey, & Parton, 1965) have been shown to be reliable (Stover & Giebink, 1967) and capable of replication (Miller, 1968). There is thus considerable support for Peterson's (1961) conclusion that "the generality of these factors appears to be enormous" (p. 206).

One of the earliest attempts to find systematic interrelationships among the psychological problems of children was the work of Luton Ackerson (1931, 1942). Using the case records of children who had been examined at the Illinois Institute for Juvenile Research between 1923 and 1927, he intercorrelated 162 descriptive characteristics for his sample of 2,113 boys and 1,181 girls. These characteristics ranged from such objective statements as "police arrest" to such inferences as "mental conflict." The examination of his intercorrelations led Ackerson to postulate the dichotomy of "personality problems" and "conduct problems," and he described the former as resulting primarily in suffering for the child, the latter in suffering for others. Lacking the statistical techniques that might have permitted a sophisticated analysis of his data, Ackerson was unable to substantiate his assertion that child behavior problems can be ordered by this dichotomous classification, but later studies tended to bear him out.

Lorr and Jenkins (1953) selected 94 of Ackerson's 162 descriptive characteristics and subjected them to a factor analysis. This resulted in the isolation of five primary factors which they labeled "socialized delinquency," "internal conflict," "unsocialized aggressiveness," "brain injury," and "schizoid pattern." These labels reflect the heterogeneity of the original Ackerson items in which several principles of classification had been confounded. Thus, "brain injury" relates to etiology, "schizoid pattern" to a severity dimension, "internal conflict" to a theoretical inference, and "socialized delinquency" to value differences between the child's immediate environment and the larger community. The only factor with a clear behavioral referent is "unsocialized aggressiveness." Since "internal conflict" is derived from such items as crying spells, sensitivity, worry, and discouraged attitudes, this factor might have been labeled more appropriately with the term "over-inhibited child" which Jenkins and Hewitt (1944) had used in an earlier publication and which would identify withdrawn behavior. Ackerson's postulated dichotomy thus seems to have some merit.

Another study in which the original Ackerson data were subjected to a factor analysis is one by Himmelweit which is cited by Eysenck (1960). Again, not all 162 items were used but, guided by theoretical assumptions about the structure of personality, only 50 were selected for study. This time three factors emerged from a factor analysis. The first, a general factor of abnormality, would seem to reflect that the data came from a disturbed population. The third factor is, according to Eysenck, "somewhat difficult to identify," but it seems to be based on items having to do with cognitive functions and work habit, items which Lorr and Jenkins (1953) had found in the factor they labeled "schizoid pattern." Of greatest interest is the bipolar second factor which distributes items along the aggression-withdrawal dimension, thus lending further support to the "personality problem-conduct problem" dichotomy originally postulated by Ackerson (1931).

Dimensions of Behavior Disorders

Unlike earlier investigators, Peterson (1961) used data uniformly gathered specifically for the purposes of his research. He thus avoided many of the problems investigators invariably encounter when they attempt *ex post facto* research on information contained in old case records. Peterson made no theoretical assumptions about the structural organization of children's behavior disorders, but the two directions that the effect of maladaptive excess behavior can take—toward the child or toward the environment—again clearly emerged.

Peterson's initial pool of problems came from the cases of a child guidance clinic and consisted of 427 items. After discarding synonymous and redundant items, he chose the 58 most frequent problems for a rating scale. This scale was submitted to 28 teachers of 831 kindergarten and elementary school children in 6 different schools. His subjects were thus not clinic cases but unselected school children, a decision which was based on the assumption that the problem behaviors seen at a clinic are continuous with general child behavior. The teachers were to rate each problem on a 3-point scale of severity, but judgments of "mild" and "severe" were later pooled for the statistical analysis. Subsequent factor analysis revealed that a 2-factor solution described the intercorrelations. Factor one was labeled "conduct problems." The items with the highest loadings on this factor, across the four age levels, were disobedience, disruptiveness, boisterousness, fighting, attention-seeking, and restlessness. The second factor was labeled "personality problems." Here the heaviest loadings were found on items describing feelings of inferiority, lack of self-confidence, social withdrawal, proneness to become flustered, self-consciousness, shyness, and anxiety.

Peterson (1961) compared mean factor scores for boys and girls across age groups and found that boys consistently displayed more "conduct problems" than girls. Younger boys also had more "personality problems," but a reversal seems to occur around the third and fourth grade, after which the scores for girls exceeded those for boys. The factor scores also showed some age-related changes in that "conduct problem" scores for both boys and girls were lower for the third and fourth grade age group than for the other three age groups. The same was true for the "personality problem" scores of boys, but the scores of girls showed a general rise. The respective relationships are shown in Figures 1 and 2.

The age-related changes in children's behavior problems are somewhat puzzling since there is no apparent reason why children in third and fourth grade should manifest fewer problems than children in lower or higher grades. Ross, Lacey and Parton (1965) analyzed the data from the standardization of their behavior checklist from this point of view but found no changes related to grade level beyond that to be expected by chance. Miller (1968) confirmed these findings in his replication study. In the absence of further research, one must assume that Peterson's results were related to

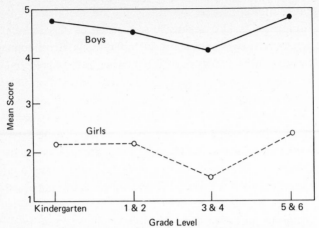

Fig. 1. Age-related changes in mean "conduct problem" scores. (After Peterson, 1961.) Copyright 1961 by the American Psychological Association and reproduced by permission.

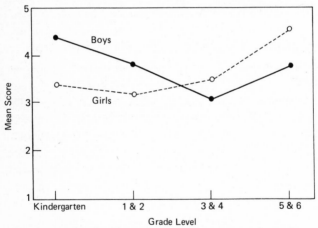

Fig. 2. Age-related changes in mean "personality problem" scores. (After Peterson, 1961.) Copyright 1961 by the American Psychological Association and reproduced by permission.

the small number of teachers used in his study. Systematic differences in teachers may well be correlated with the grade level at which they are teaching so that in responding to checklists they may be working with what Miller has called "a built-in age-correction factor." Since the environment's tolerance is part of the definition of a behavior problem, it may be that this tolerance finds expression in the way a teacher rates the behaviors found in the classroom.

Achenbach's Factor Analytic Study   The dichotomous classification of behavior disorders received further support in the research reported by Achenbach (1966). This investigator compiled a list of 91 problems and complaints (symptoms) and had raters review the case records of 300 male and 300 female children who had been referred to the child psychiatry unit of a large university hospital. Wherever a given problem was mentioned in the record, it was checked. Problems that occurred less than five times in the sample of 300 children were excluded, resulting in a final list of 74 problems. The mean number of problems recorded per case was 8.28, but this figure is biased by the fact that cases with fewer than three recordable problems had been excluded from the sample. Achenbach thus worked only with children who had multiple complaints and who had been referred to a treatment clinic. Certain other selection criteria that he used to compose the sample and that may have affected the outcome of the study should also be mentioned. There were no children with intelligence test scores of less than 75; nor were there any with serious physical illness, severe chronic physical handicap, or "good evidence for organic involvement" (p. 7). The ages ranged from four to sixteen years; all children were Caucasian, and none had been institutionalized for more than 2 years.

The data thus obtained were subjected to a factor analysis. The first principal factor that emerged for both males and females in five different analyses, and as a highly reliable dimension, was bipolar. Achenbach chose to label this factor internalizing versus externalizing and states that the problems at the externalizing pole describe "conflict with the environment," while those at the other pole describe "problems within the self" (p. 10). The nature of the problems subsumed under these two categories makes it clear that they are analogous to the "conduct problem-personality problem" dichotomy found by Peterson (1961) which in turn corresponded to the Hewitt and Jenkins (1946) terms of "unsocialized aggression" and "over-inhibited behavior," describing, in other words, aggression and withdrawal.

The second principal factor isolated in Achenbach's study was somewhat less reliable and not as readily labeled as the first. Bizarre behavior and fantastic, delusionary, or hallucinatory thinking were the two most heavily weighted problems. "Descriptively, it seemed to include symptoms both of severe mental disturbance and of excessive belligerence. The label 'Severe and Diffuse Psychopathology' was finally chosen" (p. 10). This factor bears a striking similarity to the third factor isolated by Himmelweit in the work cited by Eysenck (1960) who pointed out that it may be similar to the psychoticism factor he had identified in studies dealing with adults. The severity or intensity of a given maladaptive behavior is clearly a dimension along which psychological problems can be ordered, and factor-analytic studies help us recognize that severity is a different dimension that should not be confounded with the dimension of the direction in which excess behavior is expressed.

Because Achenbach had included certain biographical information among his data, he was able to relate this information to the internalizing and externalizing dichotomy. He found, for example, that compared to *externalizers*, the *internalizers* more frequently lived with both natural parents and that the parents had fewer overt social problems. Parents of internalizers tended to be rated as "concerned" while parents of externalizers were more frequently described as "resentful" or "indifferent." While it is somewhat hazardous to draw conclusions from these relationships because there may be a selective factor having to do with what kind of parents bring what kind of child problem to the attention of a clinic (parents of an externalizing child may be a kind who are not bothered by having an internalizing child or vice versa), Achenbach's suggestion that the socialization process plays a role in determining whether a child becomes an internalizer or externalizer has some merit. Differential reinforcement and modeling of social roles may well determine whether a child's behavior will be directed primarily against or away from the environment.

In discussing the research on the behavior of children in an unselected, nonclinic population conducted by Miller, Hampe, Barrett and Noble (1971), we mentioned that these investigators had failed to find differences between the behaviors of boys and girls, as reported by their parents. This result stands in contrast to that of Peterson (1961) whose responding teachers did record sex differences and of Achenbach (1966) whose clinic population showed sex-related differences in factor structure. After extracting his two principal factors, Achenbach subjected his data to further statistical tests. (In technical terms, he rotated the principal-factor matrix to obtain the different simple structure solutions.) Separate analyses of the data for boys and the data for girls led to the rotated factors shown in Table 1.

The order in which these factors are listed is a function of the magnitude of the factor loadings, that is, of the amount of variance accounted for by the factors. The order does not reflect the frequency with which a given problem occurred in the sample under study. It can be seen that six of these rotated factors emerge, though in different order, for boys and girls (somatic complaints, delinquent

Table 1
The Factor Structure of Disorders for Boys and for Girls*

Boys	Girls
Somatic complaints	Somatic complaints
Delinquent behavior	Delinquent behavior
Obsession, compulsions, and phobias	Obsessions, compulsions, and phobias
Sexual problems	Schizoid thinking and behavior
Schizoid thinking and behavior	Aggressive behavior
Aggressive behavior	Hyperreactive behavior
Hyperreactive behavior	Depressive symptoms
(Unnamed eighth factor)	Neurotic and delinquent behavior
	Obesity
	Anxiety symptoms
	Enuresis and other immaturities

*After Achenbach, 1966

behavior, obsessions, schizoid behavior, aggressive behavior, and hyperreactive behavior). On the other hand, the factor structure for girls is more complex, requiring eleven instead of eight factors for adequate description of the intercorrelations of the specific problems. Since the basic data used for this study were difficulties that eventuated in clinic contact, the most parsimonious explanation for this difference is that parents will bring boys to a mental health clinic for reasons that are different from those for which they will bring girls. Thus, "breathing difficulty," "excessive talking, chattering," "fainting," "inappropriate indifference, e.g., to physical complaints," "over-eating," and "picking" had been reported only for girls, while only the records of boys contained "cruelty, bullying, meanness," "fire-setting," "loudness," "sexual perversion, exposing self," "showing off," "sleepwalking," and "vandalism." These differences, which reflect differential tolerance levels on the part of society, as well as differential sex-role expectations, are the most likely reasons for the differences in factor structure. These data should not be interpreted as reflecting genetic sex-linked differences in behavior or in susceptibility to psychological disorders.

As a further aspect of his study Achenbach (1966) classified his subjects using the principal and rotated factors. Because he used the rather rigorous criterion by which a child had to have 60 percent or more of his problems come from either the internalizing or externalizing end of the first principal factor, 104 of the boys and 94 of the girls had to remain "unclassified." This approach nonetheless revealed that the children classified by the somatic, obsessive, and anxiety rotated factors fell into the internalizing category, suggesting that they had "something in common which is reflected in the functional unity of the Internalizing cluster" (p. 30). The aggressive and delinquent children, on the other hand, appeared to "have something in common which is reflected in the functional unity of the Externalizing cluster" (ibid.). The children whose problems placed them in the hyperreactive, schizoid, and depressive rotated factor classifications appeared to be less homogeneous with respect to the principal factors and did not clearly fall into either the externalizing or internalizing categories. Following his assumption that the internalizing-externalizing dimension is related to socialization, Achenbach speculates that the children in the hyperreactive, schizoid, and depressive groups may have something in common that is not directly related to the socialization dimension. While it is tempting to speculate that this "something" is related to bio-chemical, neurological, or other organic factors, such etiologi-cal questions obviously cannot be answered by factor analytic techniques.

The two directions which the immediate effect of maladaptive behavior can take, toward or away from the environment, have thus been identified as principal dimensions in a series of studies using different populations, different data sources, and different methods of analysis. They again appear in the studies still to be discussed, but here these dimensions are to be found among a number of other factors that emerged from the data analysis.

Patterson (1964) approached the classification of children with psychological problems in a manner distinctly different from the method employed in the work of Peterson (1961) or Achenbach (1966). Using a sample of 100 boys between the ages of seven and twelve years, who had intelligence test scores above 80 and were not identified as brain-injured, Patterson examined the referral problems that brought these children to three child guidance clinics. He selected thirty-nine of the most frequently occurring problems and found an average of four such problems per child. Considering this "a very inadequate sampling of the child's behav-ior" (p. 238), Patterson added 149 items based on observations made of the child's behavior during the first hour of his first clinic visit, which included some psychological testing. The behavior observations dealt with the child's appearance; his verbal, motor, and test behavior; and his approach to the interview. The 39 referral problems and 149 behavior observation items provided a correlation matrix that was then subjected to a factor analysis. Unlike the studies previously discussed, the research of Patterson thus deals primarily with a child's responses to a fairly standard stress situation, raising the question to what extent the behavior thus observed is representative of behavior away from the clinic. When, as for example in the Achenbach (1966) research, the clinical record refers to a child's disobedient, rebellious behavior, it is likely that his parents have observed this behavior in a variety of situations and over a period of time. If, on the other hand, a child upon first coming to a clinic fails to respond to the psychologist's greeting or cries during the interview, it is difficult to ascertain, as Patterson recognized, to what extent such behavior is representative of the child's day-to-day repertoire. With only 39 out of 188 variables relevant to general problem behaviors, most of the items loading on the five factors found, were items describing behavior observed in the clinic. The following factors are therefore more descriptive of the interview behavior of disturbed children than of problems around which children are brought to clinics. These considerations make it difficult to compare Patterson's work with studies previously discussed.

Factor I was given the descriptive label *hyperactive*. The most heavily loaded items on this factor suggest that it describes children who were difficult to control during psychological testing. They would issue direct commands, ask many questions, refuse to remain seated, and interrupt the tests to make comments. Among the referral problems with high loadings on this factor were "destructive" and "hyperactive, impulsive, unpredictable." While Patterson reports some consensual agreement from other psychologists with regard to the factor label, the socially oriented acting out of the children described by this factor reveals them as similar to the "conduct problem," "externalizer," or "aggression" groups of other investigators.

Factor II, which Patterson labeled *withdrawn*, clearly describes the child whom others have labeled "personality problem" or "internalizer." Factor III was labeled *immature*. Both factor and label are difficult to understand for subsumed are such items as "appropriately relaxed," "open and friendly," and "seems to enjoy test, asks for more." These would appear to be entirely adaptive behaviors, suggesting that Factor III bears some resemblance to the prosocial factor isolated by Ross, Lacey, and Parton (1965) who, in their behavior checklist, had purposely included items that might identify the well-adjusted child.

Patterson's Factor IV describes a child characterized by defensiveness and apparent tension. It is, surprisingly, labeled *aggressive* because one of the two referral problems loading high on this factor is "excessive fighting." Factor V, labeled *anxious,* derives nearly one-half of its high loading variables from the items representing referral problems. These are such complaints as obsessions and compulsions, bizarre behavior, psychosomatic symptoms, nightmares, terrors, and school phobia, suggesting that this factor identifies a severity dimension reminiscent of the second principal factor isolated by Achenbach (1966).

Taking into consideration Patterson's mixing of behavior observations with referral problems, and his somewhat idiosyncratic method of factor labeling, the dichotomy relevant to the direction of child behavior (approach or avoidance) and the dimension of severity can still be recognized.

The ambitious Behavioral Classification Project conducted under the general direction of Dreger (Dreger et al., 1964) was based on neither referral problems nor direct behavior observations but on the judgment of parents of clinic-referred children who were asked to indicate on a 229-item questionnaire whether they had observed their child engage in a given activity during the past 6 months. Although parents can be trained to be reliable observers of their child's behavior, questions requiring recall of past events on their part are likely to produce answers of questionable validity and low reliability (Robbins, 1963). Dreger's study was no exception. Interrater agreements between parents rating the same child ranged from only 10 to 55 percent with a mean of 36 percent. The questionable validity is reflected in the fact that children in a nonclinic control group were reported as engaging in proportionately more sadistic aggressiveness and social immaturity than the children referred to child guidance clinics. Because of this, the nine factors related to child behavior, derived from the intercorrelations in Dreger's study, are difficult to relate to the results of other attempts at classifying maladaptive behavior.

The conclusion that the dimensions of aggression and withdrawal have enormous generality (Peterson, 1961) when used in classifying child behavior, received further strong support from the work of Kohn (1969) who found these dimensions not only to have generality but also predictive power. Kohn (1969) administered a 90-item Social Competence Scale and a 58-item Symptom Checklist to 407 children, ranging in age from three to six, who attended day care centers operated by the welfare department of a large northeastern city. The Symptom Checklist included such items as, "Keeps to himself, remains aloof and distant," and "Gets angry or annoyed when addressed by an adult, even in friendly manner (not reprimand)." The Social Competence Scale consisted of items designed to assess the child's mastery of major areas of functioning in a preschool setting, such as "Cooperates with rules and regulations" and "Can be independent of adult in having ideas about or planning activities." This scale was so constructed that the child's functioning in five areas was covered, namely, relationship to teachers, relationship to peers, involvement in activities, self-care activities, and behavior during transitional periods. In addition to items describing high competence, such as those cited, there were items describing low competence, as for example, "Seeks adult attention by crying" or "Dawdles when required to do something."

Each child was rated by two teachers whose ratings were pooled for purposes of the factor analysis. Two bipolar factors emerged from the analysis of the Social Competence Scale. They were labeled *interest-participation* versus *apathy-withdrawal* and *cooperation-compliance* versus *anger-defiance*. These two major factors accounted for 74 percent of the total variance of the six factor solution. The factor analysis of the Symptom Checklist also revealed two major factors that accounted for a little over 50 percent of the communal variance of a nine factor solution. They were labeled *apathy-withdrawal* and *anger-defiance*.

Model Building　It will be noted that the two symptom factors in Kohn's (1969) study have the same label as the negative poles of the two social competence factors. In fact, the respective symptom factors and social competence factors had high linear correlations, reflecting that behaviors defined as low in social competence and behaviors defined as "indications of emotional disturbance" are closely related, if not identical. An item such as "Child is bossed and dominated by other children," which appears on the Social Competence Scale, is clearly another version of "Withdraws or accepts it when others shove, hit, accuse or criticize him" which appears on the Symptom Checklist. It would seem that an assessment of social competence permits one to classify children into four major groupings, as indicated in the quadrants of Figure 3. The left column identifies children whose behavior is considered adaptive, while the right column identifies those whose behavior is considered maladaptive—society having defined defiance of norms and withdrawal from social interaction as negative or deviant behaviors.

Such a fourfold classification of behavior was suggested by Schaefer (1961) when he advanced his hypothetical "circumplex model" for social and emotional behavior, which was arranged around the orthogonal axes of extraversion-introversion and hostility-love. Schaefer (1961) identified the resulting four combinations of these dimensions as "friendliness—outgoing, positive behavior; conformity—compliant, controlled positive behavior; withdrawal—hostile, fearful avoidance of interaction, and aggressiveness—hostile attack with little impulse control" (p. 139). The results of Kohn's (1969) large-scale study would seem to support these four combinations, if not to confirm Schaefer's hypothetical model.

Kohn's work (1969) is of particular interest because it extends the classification of behavior to a younger age group and into the adaptive realm whereas earlier work had dealt almost exclusively with maladaptive behavior of older children. Kohn also reports a highly important follow-up study which revealed that the factors

Activity Level	Behavior Judged Positive (Adaptive)	Behavior Judged Negative (Maladaptive)
Active	Interest - Participation	Anger - Defiance
Passive	Cooperation - Compliance	Apathy - Withdrawal

Fig. 3.   A fourfold classification of social competence. (Based on Kohn, 1969.)

have stability and predictive power. One hundred of the children who had been rated in the original study were reevaluated in their first year in public school, using the Metropolitan Achievement Test and Peterson's problem checklist. It was found that children who had been high on apathy-withdrawal in preschool scored high on Peterson's analogous "personality problem" factor, while children who had scored high on anger-defiance scored high on Peterson's analogous "conduct problem" factor. The significant product-moment correlations were .22 and .40, respectively. This indicates, as Kohn (1969) points out, that these children continued to display behaviors in first grade that are similar to those they had exhibited earlier in the pre-school day care center, despite changes in school and teachers. One can thus conclude with reasonable confidence that aggression and withdrawal are behavioral characteristics that permit a reliable and predictively valid mode of classifying the behavior of children whether they are found in special treatment clinics or in the general population. This, in turn, confirms that the behavior of disturbed children is not qualitatively different from the behavior of so-called normal children; the behavior lies on the same continuum, and only a judgment of magnitude (too much or too little), which is a function of the tolerance level of the people who make the judgment, separates the child in the clinic from the child in the school. This conclusion was also reached by Miller, Hampe, Barrett, and Noble (1971) in their survey of children's deviant behavior within the general population. If maladaptive behavior is simply that behavior which society has labeled maladaptive and is thus behavior that follows the same principles of development and change as any other form of behavior, a meaningful classificatory system must reflect this continuity.

Based on this logic, Becker and Krug (1964) proposed a circumplex model for the social behavior of children. Working, in part, with data from an earlier study (Becker, Peterson, Luria, Shoemaker, & Hellmer, 1962) which were derived from behavior ratings on five-year-old children, Becker and Krug (1964) graphically plotted the positions of five bipolar variables, generating the model shown in Figure 4. The generality of this approach was tested by assigning the results of studies by six different investigators to this

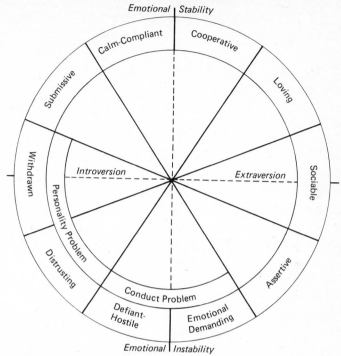

Fig. 4. A circumplex model of child behavior. (After Becker and Krug, 1964.) Copyright 1964 by The Society for Research in Child Development and reproduced by permission.

circumplex. High concordance was demonstrated in this manner, reflecting the meaningfulness of the approach and its utility in ordering data on child behavior. As can be seen from the accompanying figure, the model incorporates the stability-instability and introversion-extraversion factors, and it also identifies the location of the "personality problem" and "conduct problem" sectors previously identified by Peterson (1961). The similarity between the active-passive and positive-negative categories shown in Figure 3 to the introversion-extraversion and stability-instability dimensions in Figure 4 reflects the fact that a number of classificatory schemes of similar merit are possible and that the labeling of dimensions is a function of a given author's personal or theoretical preferences.

The fact that descriptions of child behavior lend themselves to categorizations that can be represented in two-dimensional drawings should not lead one to lose sight of the fact that these dimensions are not dimensions of child behavior but dimensions of adults' reports of child behavior. This distinction was stressed by Novick, Rosenfeld, Bloch, and Dawson (1966) who very correctly point out that one must distinguish between reports on behavior and the behavior actually emitted by the child. This becomes particularly crucial when the reports use categories requiring the respondent to draw inferences and make generalizations. If, as was the case in the study by Becker et al. (1962), the parent or teacher is required to rate children on such dimensions as "dominant-submissive" or "soft-hearted–hard-hearted," the rating may say more about the respondent's perception than the child's behavior. Even where one can get high interobserver reliability on a rating of "dominant" for a given child, it would seem likely that the child is dominant in some situations and vis-a-vis certain peers but submissive under different conditions.

What emerges is the importance of maintaining a focus on objectively observable behavior while spelling out the stimulus conditions under which this behavior is observed. When this is done, as was the case in the work of Kohn (1969), for example, a model like the one proposed by Becker and Krug (1964) can serve the useful function of ordering the data and conceptualizing the relationship between response classes.

RECAPITULATION

The definition of psychological disorders suggested in Chapter 1 speaks of behavior that deviates from the social norm in that it occurs with a frequency or intensity that the child's social environment deems either too high or too low. We pointed out that one can thus speak of deficient behavior and of excess behavior and that within these classes one can distinguish a variety of categories. Excess behavior, we said, can take two forms: excessive approach responses or excessive avoidance responses; the former often being called "aggressive," the latter "withdrawn" behavior.

The results of the factor analytic studies reviewed in the

preceding pages would seem to lend strong support to the assumption that this is indeed a useful way of classifying disorders which are characterized by excess behavior. On the other hand, these studies have lent very little, if any, support to the notion that there is another major class of behavior disorders which might be placed in the rubric of deficient behavior. The reason for this can be traced back to the decisions an investigator must make when he plans a factor analytic study of behavior disorders.

One of the decisions, made by investigator after investigator, is to limit his sample to children with intelligence test scores in the normal range and without known brain injury. Achenbach (1966), for example, excluded children with intelligence test scores below 75 and "good evidence for organic involvement," while Patterson (1964) required that the children in his sample had intelligence test scores above 80 and that they had not been identified as brain-injured. Such a selection would obviously bias the data in such a way that it would be surprising to find a factor representing behaviors that are characteristic of children who are inadequate in the area of intellectual functioning.

Another decision in research strategy that would work against the emergence of factors reflecting deficient behavior is to study children being observed at child guidance clinics or to use an item pool derived from complaints about children's social behavior found in the records of such clinics. In the 20 years between 1946 and 1966, when all of the studies we have reviewed were conducted, community child guidance clinics operated in a tradition that defined mental subnormality as an area outside the interest and competence of the professional staff of such clinics. Retarded children were rarely referred to them, and if such a child did find his way to their door, he would be quickly sent elsewhere because his problems were deemed not amenable to the form of treatment (psychotherapy) these clinics were then dispensing (Ross, 1959).

A similar selection bias militates against the emergence of a factor that might identify the grossly atypical behavior of the autistic child. *Early infantile autism*, a condition we shall discuss here under the heading deficient behavior, occurs so rarely that data gathered from either child guidance records or from a sample of the general population will not result in a factor structure where the behaviors of the autistic child can receive sufficient loading to be recognized.

Juvenile delinquency is another heading in the section of this book which deals with deficient behavior. This, as we shall attempt to explain, derives from the formulation of the problems of the so-called delinquent as being primarily in the area of deficient self-control over unacceptable behavior. We shall also point out that juvenile delinquency is not a psychological entity but a judicial label, and so it is not surprising that factor-analytic studies of child behavior have rarely led to a factor that can be labeled *delinquency*. The items identifying this behavior have usually emerged under such labels as "conduct problems" or "unsocialized aggressiveness" and only once (Lorr & Jenkins, 1953) as "socialized delinquency." The fact that only the data originally gathered by Ackerson (1931) eventuated in a delinquency factor when subjected to a factor analysis by Lorr and Jenkins points to another instance of the operation of a selection bias. Most child guidance clinics saw very few juvenile delinquents in the two decades which furnished the data for the factor analytic studies. The delinquents' problems were viewed as of a different order from the "emotionally disturbed" child favored by these clinics, largely because it had been found that their treatment was ineffective when used with a delinquent population. Ackerson's data, however, were collected before that period, during a time when the Chicago Institute for Juvenile Research (where his data were gathered) was still accepting delinquents, for whose study and treatment it had, in fact, been specifically created.

There remains the question why learning difficulties, clearly a behavior deficit, did not show up in most factor-analytic studies. The answer can again be found in the decisions investigators make in the course of planning, conducting, and interpreting a factor-analytic study. Ross, Lacey, and Parton (1965) chose to exclude any item that referred to a child's academic performance in order to avoid a negative halo effect in the teachers' ratings. This decision obviously made it impossible for a learning disability factor to emerge. When Miller (1967b) modified that checklist by adding school-performance items, he did indeed find a factor which was labeled *learning disabilities.* In Peterson's (1961) work, items related to school performance, such as inattentiveness, laziness in school, shortness of attention span, and distractibility had approximately equal, low factor loadings on both the "conduct problem" and the "personality problem" factors; a different statistical strategy might well have resulted in the emergence of a factor related to school performance. Still another reason for the rare emergence of a learning disability factor lies in the arbitrariness of factor labeling. As was pointed out earlier, the factor Lorr and Jenkins (1953) chose to label "schizoid pattern" is derived from items dealing with cognitive functions and work habits, items for which this label seems quite inappropriate.

For purposes of organizing the psychological disorders to be discussed in chapters to follow, it seemed heuristically desirable to speak of *deficient behavior* and *excess behavior* and to place the discussion of learning difficulties under the former rubric, together with the categories early infantile autism, mental subnormality, juvenile delinquency, and psychophysiologic disorders. Aggressive behavior, withdrawn behavior, and psychotic disorders, on the other hand, will be found under the overall heading *excess behavior* for reasons which will hopefully become clear from the discussions found in the respective chapters.

3

CONSTITUTIONAL FACTORS IN BEHAVIORAL STYLE

Careful students of child behavior (Irwin, 1930; Shirley, 1933) have long ago reported striking individual differences in the behavioral style of very young children. Activity level, motility, frequency of crying, amount of food intake, and the sleep-wake cycle are among the many characteristics in which differences seem to be present from the time of birth. Lately it has come to be recognized that these early individual differences contribute importantly to the organism-environment interaction which eventuates in that complex behavioral repertoire of the individual that we sometimes call personality. More specifically, it would seem to be a reasonable hypothesis that individual differences in behavioral style, interacting with the social environment, are an important factor in the development of behavior disorders.

> From the infant's first day of life on, a mother and her child are each unique individuals. Their responses to each other are based on their respective reaction patterns (personalities) within the matrix of the total environmental situation obtaining at the time. . . Any particular mother will react to a child

with a high activity level in a different manner than to a child with a low activity level [Ross, 1959, p. 76].

The potential stress resulting from a mismatch between the mother's expectations or tolerances and the child's behavioral style may well set the stage for discord and conflict.

In terms of Cattell's (1950) "three modalities of behavior traits," the largely constitutional behavioral style is the quality in which behavior finds expression; it is the *how* of behavior, as opposed to the *why* (motivation) and the *what* (abilities and content). Like other constitutional *Anlagen* (predispositions), behavioral style can be modified within limits by environmental influences; it is not an immutable characteristic, but it is well to keep in mind that the ultimate behavioral outcome is the consequence of influences on an already existing style, not the result of the environment shaping a tabula rasa child. Strong support for this formulation was presented by Schaefer and Bayley (1963) who analyzed the extensive collection of longitudinal data from the Berkeley Growth Study and found that the child dimension of activity-passivity was relatively independent of parent-child relationships. They viewed this finding as supporting the hypothesis that the human infant is not completely plastic but responds to his environment in accordance with his innate tendencies.

The behavioral point of view which represents the basic orientation of this book risks giving the impression that environmental factors are solely responsible for the development of behavior. This impression can arise from the fact that we manipulate environmental factors when we seek to modify behavior, but, as was stressed in the Introduction, one must not conclude that only environmental factors were responsible for the development of a given behavior merely because that behavior can be modified by working only on these factors. It is as yet one more attempt to avert that *post hoc, ergo propter hoc* fallacy that the following material on behavioral style is presented before a discussion of psychological disorders.

BEHAVIORAL INDIVIDUALITY IN EARLY CHILDHOOD

The most systematic approach to the question of behavioral style and its contribution to child development is the work of Thomas, Chess, and Birch (1968) who carried out a longitudinal study of 136 children with a focus on behavioral individuality in early childhood (Thomas, Chess, Birch, Hertzig, & Korn, 1963). Without claiming that their sample is representative of the general population (the mean Stanford-Binet IQ of the children was 127), these investigators present a framework for the discussion of behavioral style that has far-reaching implications for the student of psychological disorders of children.

The study extended over a 10-year period during which data-gathering entailed parental interviews, teacher interviews, school observations, and observations of the child in the course of individual intelligence testing. The mean age of the children at the time of the first parental interview was 3.3 months, 50 percent of them being less than 2.5 months old. Parental interviews were repeated at 3-month intervals during the first 18 months; they were then held at intervals of 6 months until the child was five years old; thereafter interviews were held on a yearly basis. School observations of one hour and teacher interviews began when the child entered nursery school and were repeated each year. The Stanford-Binet, Form L was administered at ages three and six. In addition to the regular parental interviews, a special structured interview was held with each parent separately when the child was three years old. Validity of the information elicited from the parents was checked by independent observers who went to the homes of 23 of the 136 children. Throughout the study the investigators used reasonable safeguards against confounding the data by using interviewers and observers who had no knowledge of the child's previous history or behavior. The reliability of interview and observation scoring is adequate for purposes of an investigation of this type (Thomas et al., 1963).

Throughout the interviews with parents and teachers the focus was on factual descriptions of actual behavior, and inferences as to the "meaning" of the behavior were not accepted. Thus, when a parent reported that the child "loved his cereal," the interviewer had been instructed to inquire what specific aspect of the child's behavior made the parent come to this conclusion. Individual patterns of behavioral style seemed to emerge particularly around the child's reaction to new stimuli, demands, or situations —whether these were simple, as the first bath, or complex, as entry into nursery school. For this reason, special attention was paid to the child's first response to a new stimulus and to his subsequent reactions when the same stimulus was again presented.

Temperamental Characteristics

An inductive content analysis of the parental interviews for the first twenty-two children studied led the investigators to establish the following nine categories of behavioral style, called *temperamental characteristics* by the authors (Thomas et al., 1963).

ACTIVITY LEVEL   This refers to the level, tempo, and frequency of general motility. A child with high activity level is described as wriggling, kicking, moving, squirming, and running around a great deal. Parents would make such comments as: "He crawls all over the house," "He runs around so, that whenever we come in from the park I'm exhausted," or "He moves a great deal in his sleep." Low activity level, on the other hand, was described as: "In the bath he lies quietly and doesn't kick" or "In the morning he's still in the same place he was when he fell asleep." The characteristic of activity level was rated on a 3-point scale, could be reliably identified, and showed consistency over time. The same was true of all temperamental characteristics.

RHYTHMICITY   This category reflects the degree of regularity of such repetitive biological functions as sleeping and waking, rest and activity, as well as the food intake and elimination cycles. Scoring was based on the regularity or irregularity of these events.

APPROACH OR WITHDRAWAL   The initial reaction of the child to any new stimulus, such as food, toys, people, places, or procedures, can be categorized along this dimension on the basis of parental report and observations. "He always smiles at a stranger" is an example of the approach reaction, while "Whenever he sees a stranger he cries" describes a child whose preponderant style is to withdraw.

ADAPTABILITY   While the preceding category referred to the initial response, adaptability deals with the modifiability of the initial pattern, that is, with the sequential course of responses to new situations. Inasmuch as parents tend to view initial withdrawal or negative responses as changeworthy, adaptive behavior is likely to be required to the demands of the social environment. Thus, the child who spat out the cereal when it was first fed to him but who later came to accept it with little protest is considered adaptable, while the one who continues to reject the food manifests nonadaptive behavior. Thomas, Chess, and Birch (1968) present excerpts from parental interviews to illustrate this behavioral characteristic. Thus, "Now when we go to the doctor's he doesn't start to cry till we undress him, and he even stops then if he can hold a toy." As an example of nonadaptive behavior they reproduce the following statement: "Whenever I put his snowsuit and hat on he screams and struggles, and he doesn't stop crying till we're outside."

INTENSITY OF REACTION   Whether a response is negative or positive, it can be emitted with high or low intensity, and each child has a dominant characteristic on this dimension that tends to run across modalities and situations. Intensity was scored in relation to responses to external stimuli as well as to deprivation and satiation. An example of high-intensity reaction is "He cries loud and long whenever the sun shines in his eyes," of low intensity, "He squints at a bright light but doesn't cry."

THRESHOLD OF RESPONSIVENESS This category deals with the intensity of the stimulus that is required in order to elicit an observable response. Threshold may differ for different sensory systems so that a child can have a high threshold for visual but a low threshold for auditory stimuli. Subsumed under this category is the concept of difference in limen, the magnitude of difference between stimuli necessary before the child shows evidence of discrimination. For example, "He notices any little change."

QUALITY OF MOOD This category differentiates between the child whose pervasive mood is friendly, pleasant, and joyful ("He always smiles at a stranger") and the child who tends to behave in a generally unfriendly, unpleasant manner ("He cries at almost every stranger, and those that he doesn't cry at he hits"). Positive mood tends to manifest itself in smiling and laughing, while negative mood is characterized by frowning and crying. As with all other categories, scoring is based on observable behavior, not on inferred states of unhappiness or happiness.

DISTRACTIBILITY This category was used to indicate the ease or difficulty with which ongoing behavior can be interrupted by extraneous environmental stimuli. These stimuli may be introduced by a parent who desires to distract a child from an undesirable activity, or they may be chance stimuli in the environment that draw the child's attention from an ongoing activity.

ATTENTION SPAN AND PERSISTENCE Attention span refers to the length of time a given activity is pursued, while persistence involves the question whether an activity is maintained despite interruptions and other obstacles. Although distractibility and persistence would seem to be reciprocal, it is necessary to treat them as separate categories because it is possible for a child to be both highly distractible and highly persistent. Such a child would return to a given task again and again, no matter how often he is distracted or diverted.

As might be expected, these nine categories of behavioral style are interrelated. This interrelationship is reflected in correlations ranging from $-.49$ to $+.48$. The largest number of significant correlations with other categories was found for intensity, adaptability, and mood quality; the interrelations among the other categories were low and generally insignificant. A factor analysis of the nine categories for each of the first 5 years of the subject's life revealed a clustering of mood, intensity, approach-withdrawal, and adaptability on the first factor of a varimax solution. The loadings on this factor range from $.34$ to $.77$; the loadings on the other two factors that emerged were considerably lower, and the clusters made little theoretical sense. The first factor, labeled Factor A, was thus selected for further use, to be discussed below.

Behavioral Style and Psychological Disorders
Of the 136 children in the study, 42 were identified as manifesting psychological disorders in the course of the 10-year contact with the research team. Children with psychological disorders thus represented 31 percent of the total study population. This figure denotes the prevalence of disorders over a 10-year span and is thus higher than the usually reported incidence data which are based on cross-sectional surveys at one point in time. Nonetheless, it is likely that the families' ongoing contact with the research team, the availability of a child psychiatrist on the team, the recurrent interviews which were focused on child behavior, and the general level of sophistication of these parents resulted in their seeking help with problem behaviors more readily and earlier than might be expected of parents in the general population.

To be included in the so-called clinical sample, a child had to manifest disordered behavior which the team's child psychiatrist judged as representing a significant behavioral disturbance. Most (86 percent) of the children in the clinical sample were designated as manifesting mild or moderate reactive behavior disorders, such as sleep problems, peer difficulties, tantrums, or learning difficulties—complaints quite similar to those usually encountered by child guidance clinics. For all of these cases parental guidance was the recommended form of treatment, reflecting, as we shall see, the orientation of the study team.

Since in all but one of the forty-two cases it was the parents' complaint about the child's behavior which was instrumental in initiating the psychiatric study, it is of interest to examine the kind of behaviors the parents considered problematic. As Thomas et al. (1968) point out, these closely reflect current child-care practices, expressing standards and attitudes prevalent among the total study sample. The parents were relatively tolerant of difficulties in the areas of eating, elimination, and masturbation which, though they reported them in the interviews, they did not define as problems. They tended to complain more about disturbances in the areas of sleep, discipline, and mood; but the greatest frequency of complaints occurred in the areas of speech difficulties, peer relationships, and school learning. Thus it appears that the more readily a difficulty is visible to the outside world, the more readily the parents in this group defined it as a problem and sought help. Whatever functions are high in the value hierarchy of parents will become important considerations affecting the parent-child interaction by defining the focus of parental concern with selected aspects of the child's behavior. The presenting complaints encountered by the clinician may thus reflect current parental values and attitudes at least as much as the adaptive difficulties prevalent in the child population at any given time.

The availability of the independently assessed data on behavioral style enabled the research team to make various comparisons between the temperamental characteristics of their clinical and nonclinical samples. The forty-two clinical cases had been further subdivided into children with "active" disturbances (n = 34) and children with "passive" disturbances (n = 8). The characteristic

behavior of the children in the passive group was their nonpartici-
pation in peer group activities. If the child displayed any behavior
such as crying or running away or if he had physical complaints,
such as nausea or stomach pains, he was regarded as a child with
active disturbance.

Comparison between the nonclinical group and the children
with active disturbances revealed that the latter had received
significantly higher scores on activity level in their first year of life.
Other variables of behavioral style such as intensity, adaptability,
threshold, distractibility, and persistence were significantly different
at later ages. The comparison between children with passive problems and the nonclinical group did not reveal early differences; but
by the fourth and fifth year of life the children with passive problems were significantly more negative in mood, less active, more
persistent, and more withdrawing in response to new stimuli than
the nonclinical contrast group.

It should be recalled that a factor analysis based on the intercorrelations of the nine categories of behavioral style had identified a
factor, labeled Factor A, that had high loadings on mood, intensity,
approach-withdrawal, and adaptability and showed relative consistency over the first 5-year period. Comparison between the clinical groups (active and passive) and the nonclinical group revealed
that over the 5-year period and starting around the third year the
clinical group came to deviate markedly from the nonclinical group
in the direction of negative mood, marked intensity, and tendency
to withdraw and to be nonadaptive.

Taking only those children who had been referred because of
active problem behaviors before age five and comparing these on the
nine categories and on Factor A with children in the nonclinical
group, Thomas and his coworkers found that for each of the
comparisons and for at least 4 of the 5 years, the children with
behavior disorders deviated in temperament in the direction signi-
fying greater adaptational difficulty. Particularly for Factor A, the
clinical group differed from the nonclinical group in the nonadaptive
direction in every one of the 5 years, becoming increasingly
deviant over time. These findings suggest that children who come
to be referred to a clinic *before they are five years old* tend to differ

from children who, over a 10-year period, are never referred in the characteristics of mood, intensity, approach-withdrawal, and adaptability. The investigators took pains to point out that a given combination of behavioral styles in a specific child does not in and of itself lead to behavior problems but that it is the interaction between these stylistic characteristics and the child's environment which can eventuate in clinical referral.

It is important to recognize that behavioral style and environment not only interact but that they also modify each other and that the child's behavior has as much of an effect on his parents' actions as their behavior has on his (Yarrow, Waxler, & Scott, 1971). The child's behavioral style clearly represents a stimulus constellation to which his parents respond and that response, in turn, may be a function of the parents' behavioral style. On the basis of their observations, Thomas et al. (1963) conclude that life experiences can modify a child's behavioral style. Repeatedly faced with his parents' impossible demands, a child who is initially very adaptable can become increasingly less adaptable over time. As with other behavioral styles, a child with a high score on adaptability is a child who is predominantly but not universally adaptive. Repeated negative experiences can result in a change in the ratio of adaptive to maladaptive response patterns. It is further possible that as the child gets older, he comes to recognize that certain aspects of his behavioral style tend to have negative consequences so that he may learn to modify or control some of his reactions under certain circumstances.

Difficult Children

The interaction between behavioral style and environment is most readily illustrated by tracing the experiences of some of the children with a behavioral style marked by irregularity, nonadaptability, withdrawal responses, and predominantly negative moods of high intensity—a constellation which characterizes what Thomas and his colleagues chose to call "difficult children." Irregularity of biological functions may find expression in the areas of sleeping, eating, and elimination. As infants, these children will wake up at unpredictable intervals and seem to require less sleep than the average child of the same age. Since they do not develop regular sleep cycles, these infants' parents are awakened several times a night, and no matter what techniques they might try, they will find it impossible to get the child to sleep through the night. Similar unpredictability can be found in the irregularity with which hunger is expressed. The amount of food consumed at any given time and the intervals between eating can vary greatly, making it impossible for the mother to work out a self-demand schedule. Unpredictable preferences for specific foods which may undergo abrupt changes can also characterize these children, much to the exasperation of their parents. With similar unpredictability of elimination cycles, toilet-training procedures that are based on the parent's ability to anticipate the child's eliminations are doomed to failure.

The temperamental tendency of these children to withdraw in the face of new stimuli is particularly obvious in early infancy when new experiences are constantly impinging on the child. These children are described as crying when bathed for the first time, crying whenever a new food is introduced, and crying whenever a new person enters the room. Leaving the house may result in crying, protesting, clinging, and withdrawing, with the same reactions being evoked when returning to the house at the end of an excursion. The predominance of high-intensity negative mood is manifested by relatively more crying than laughing, more fussing than expressions of pleasure.

It should by now be apparent why Thomas, Chess, and Birch labeled these as "difficult children." A child with these temperamental characteristics places special demands on his parents, and their reactions will play a major role in determining the course of the child's behavioral development.

The longitudinal data available to Thomas and his coworkers enable one to contrast the development of two of these "difficult children," thereby demonstrating the crucial role of parental reaction patterns. Both children, one a girl, the other a boy, displayed similar behavioral characteristics in the early years of life. They had irregular sleep patterns, difficulty with bowel movements, slow acceptance of new foods, lengthy periods of adjustment to new routines, and frequent periods of loud crying. The girl's father reacted to her behavior with anger, seemed to dislike the child, and spent little or no time with her. The mother, on the other hand, was more understanding and permissive but quite inconsistent. The only rules that were consistently enforced were those involving the child's safety. Both the father and the mother of the boy, on the other hand, were unusually tolerant and consistent. They accepted his lengthy periods of adaptation patiently and calmly and reacted to his negative moods without anger. They viewed his troublesome behavior as an expression of his individual characteristics and not as indications of a behavioral disturbance. By age five and a half the boy was functioning smoothly in peer relations and nursery school activity. By this time, the girl manifested explosive outbursts of anger, soiling, thumbsucking, fear of the dark, protective lying, negativism, poor peer relationships, and an insatiable demand for toys and candy.

It may well be that casual acceptance of temperamental characteristics permits a child to adapt at his own pace to the demands of his environment. On the other hand, the reaction which makes each incident into a conflict is likely to reinforce that particular behavioral characteristic, giving the previously innate pattern an operant quality which strengthens and thus perpetuates it.

Compared to the children with easier temperamental characteristics, the "difficult children" were far less likely to grow up without behavior problems. Approximately 70 percent of the temperamentally difficult children are reported as having developed such problems. Difficult children represented 23 percent of the total clinical group of forty-two but only 4 percent of the nonclinical sample. It is a challenging research question whether the incidence of behavior disorders among "difficult children" can be reduced by educating parents to accept their child's individuality and helping them to adapt to his behavioral style so that the child in turn can adapt to the successive demands of socialization.

The orientation of the clinical and research group working with Thomas permitted them to focus on manifest behavior in working with the cases in the clinical group. In the majority of these cases the choice of treatment was parent guidance focused on environmental changes and modification of parental functioning in dealing with the child. The interviews concentrated on the need for the parents to recognize and accept their child's individual pattern of behavioral style. The parents were advised to desist from unrealistic attempts to change the child's characteristic reaction patterns. With an older child it was sometimes possible to acquaint him with his own temperamental characteristics and to teach him ways of arranging situations so as to minimize the negative consequences of his behavioral characteristics. When a child knows, for example, that he characteristically has intense negative reactions to new situations, he can learn to introduce himself into such situations gradually, thereby reducing his negative reactions that may otherwise give him trouble. Thomas, Chess, and Birch view the reality of individual behavioral style not as an inevitability that must be fatalistically accepted but as a condition which, once recognized, gives both parent and child logical means of coping with individual differences.

RECAPITULATION

In discussing the determinants of behavior in the Introduction to this book, we stressed that one of the four interacting factors which enter into any specific behavior is the genetic-constitutional characteristic of the individual. The present chapter contains a summary of an important research project that has attempted to isolate some of these characteristics with particular reference to their role in the development of behavior disorders. The work of Thomas, Chess, and Birch (1968) has its limitations, particularly in terms of sampling, but whether or not it can be considered definitive, it should serve as a reminder that the child makes an important contribution to the interaction with his environment. This contribution consists, among other things, of such behavioral style characteristics as activity level, rhythmicity of biological functions, approach or withdrawal reactions to new stimuli, adaptability, intensity of reaction, threshold of responsiveness, mood quality, distractibility, attention span, and persistence. Depending on his particular combination of these characteristics, parents may find the child easy or difficult to take care of, and "difficult children" may be contributing more than their share to the psychological disorders to be discussed in the pages to follow.

PART II

DEFICIENT BEHAVIOR

4

EARLY INFANTILE AUTISM

There is a great deal of confusion in the professional literature about the use of the word *autism.* In its original sense, autism refers to a distorted, self-centered form of thinking that is controlled by the thinker's needs or desires and bears little relation to external reality; the form of thinking which takes place in dreams, daydreams, and fantasy. As such, autism is a normal phenomenon, provided the person who engages in such thinking is able to differentiate between reality and fantasy and as long as autistic distortions of reality do not come to control the person's behavior. When an individual acts on the basis of his autistic productions—taking them, as it were, for his perception of reality—he becomes unable to cope adaptively with the demands of his environment; his behavior would then be classified as *psychotic.* The profoundly disordered, psychotic child probably engages in autistic thinking; yet, the term *autistic child* is not synonymous with psychotic child. To reduce the possible confusion, the term autism, in the context of disturbed behavior, should be used only when it is intended to refer to that highly specific and quite rare form of profoundly disordered behavior whose full technical name is *early infantile autism.*

Early infantile autism was first described and named by Leo Kanner (1943) who, in his psychiatric practice, had encountered a small number of children who displayed a cluster of behaviors that made them appear to belong to a unique group. While Kanner's medical orientation led him to view this behavior cluster as a syndrome defining a disease entity, there is, at this point, no reliable psychometric evidence to support the existence of such an entity. As Masters and Miller (1970) have pointed out, there has, as yet, been no valid, empirical demonstration of early infantile autism as anything more than a nonobservable construct based on a hypothesized interrelationship among observable events. These observable events characterize the group of children who fall in the rubric of early infantile autism, and one can discuss these behavioral characteristics without assuming that they define a disease entity.

CHARACTERISTICS OF THE AUTISTIC CHILD

As its name implies, early infantile autism occurs in a child's early infancy, and parents usually report that their child displayed behavior deficits and was "different" from the moment of birth. They recall that the child failed to anticipate being picked up and that he reacted as if other people did not exist. As the child gets older, this *autistic aloneness* takes the form of an absence of interpersonal behavior. He does not emit the social smile, seems not to recognize members of his family, and does not engage in such social games as peek-a-boo or pat-a-cake. He will fail to develop appropriate language; a deficiency or gross distortion of speech for purposes of communication is one of the most frequently reported characteristics of autistic children. Another, is their pronounced insistence on sameness, coupled with a stereotyped preoccupation with a limited number of inanimate objects to which they often cling with great tenacity. Despite these marked behavior deviations, medical examinations reveal no gross neurological impairment, and the child's physical development usually proceeds normally.

When Ward (1970) reviewed the available literature, he found that the above characteristics are generally agreed upon as defining early infantile autism although, as we shall see, there continues to be much disagreement regarding the etiology of this condition—if indeed it is *a* condition in the sense of being a unitary behavior disorder that can be reliably discriminated from other profound disturbances in child behavior.

Children who display all four of the characteristics just presented—early onset of autistic aloneness, absence or distortion of language, stereotyped insistence on sameness, and lack of demonstrable physical defect—are exceedingly rare. It has been estimated that less than 1 percent of the clinic population in a large child psychiatric center meets the criteria for being appropriately called cases of early infantile autism (Kanner, 1958). Careless usage of this term has led to its application to children who manifest profound behavior deviations without meeting the necessary defining characteristics, and this has contributed to confounding the issue and complicating needed research. Until there is general agreement among clinicians and research investigators as to what children to include in a given category, little progress can be expected.

Despite its rarity, early infantile autism has attracted a great deal of clinical and scientific interest, largely on the assumption that detailed study of grossly deviant development might lead to a better understanding of the principles underlying normal development (Sarason & Gladwin, 1958). For example, the language peculiarity of autistic children raises the question how children, in general, acquire the appropriate use of pronouns. The few autistic children who develop language frequently manifest *pronominal reversal*; they will repeat personal pronouns the way they hear them, thus speaking of themselves as "you" and of the person addressed as "I." A moment's reflection on how difficult it is to try and correct a child who speaks in this manner ("No, you should not say you, you should say I") highlights the as yet unanswered question of how normal children master the correct usage of I and you. Whether the study of deviant development will indeed contribute to an understanding of normal development is, of course, a question only the future can answer. It would seem more logical to expect that the proper study of normal development is normal development and to assume that full understanding of normal processes will permit the prediction and control (understanding) of deviant processes. Be that as it may, infantile autism presents enough of a problem in its own right to warrant study for its own sake and for the sake of the children whose grossly deviant behavior gets them placed in this category.

ETIOLOGICAL SPECULATIONS

Early infantile autism has been attributed to a wide variety of causes, ranging from strictly environmental (Ferster, 1961) to purely constitutional (Rimland, 1964), with interactional formulations (Zaslow & Breger, 1969) taking the middle ground. Each of these positions points to a treatment approach that is logically consistent with the causal speculations, and positive results reported with the treatment approach are often taken as support for the causal speculation.

The logical fallacy in this reasoning should be recognized before we take a look at some representative theorizing. The fact that one can modify a given maladaptive behavior through the application of principles of operant conditioning, for example, does not provide proof that these principles were operating when the maladaptive behavior originally developed. The only way a causal sequence can ever become known is to trace the development of a disorder from its onset on the basis of careful and complete longitudinal observations on a large enough number of cases to permit the generalization that all cases of this nature develop in this way. Retrospective reconstruction, based on mothers' recalls of the events in their children's earliest days, has been shown to possess neither reliability (Wenar, 1961) nor validity (Robbins, 1963). Nor is the demonstration that isolated "autistic" behavior, such as head banging, can be shaped in monkeys through operant techniques (Schaefer, 1970) more than a provocative analogue.

Ultimately, speculations about etiology are by nature theoretical and theories can never be proven, in the sense that they can be shown to be true or false. Theories are only as good as their capacity to order available facts and to permit the generation of testable hypotheses; it is by these criteria that the following formulations should be judged.

Operant Reinforcement

The most detailed statement of a purely environmentalist hypothesis about the development of early infantile autism is that presented by Ferster (1961) who uses infantile autism as synonymous with "childhood schizophrenia" which, in turn, he views as a prototype of adult schizophrenia. Despite this rather idiosyncratic terminology, Ferster's description of the children he discusses makes it clear that he is talking about early infantile autism, as usually defined.

Ferster examines the major characteristics of the autistic child's behavior from the standpoint of functional analysis which leads him to ask what specific effects the child's behavior has on his environment and how these effects maintain his behavior. He observes that the behavioral repertoire of the autistic child is limited and that the absolute amount of his activity is low. In fact, he believes that the principal difference between the autistic child and the normal child is in the relative frequency of behavior. The major performance deficit of the autistic child, according to Ferster, lies in the degree to which his behavior is a function of the behavior of others. He points out that the limited speech of the autistic child is not maintained by its effect on the social environment; it does not benefit the listener (as would the communication of a descriptive statement) but results in immediate benefit to the speaker (as does a statement of a demand). When the child's behavior has an effect on his environment, it usually does so because the behavior is an aversive stimulus for others. This is the case with such atavisms as tantrums and self-destructive, self-mutilating behavior which often occur at relatively high frequency. The rest of the autistic child's performance is of a simple sort, having only slight effect on the environment, such as finger flipping, twisting soft objects, or rubbing a smooth surface. The strongest reinforcing stimuli are food, candy, or ice cream while secondary reinforcers are weak, and generalized reinforcers, such as a smile or adult approval, seem to maintain little of the autistic child's behavior.

The range of responses and of effective reinforcers is thus severely limited. Equally minimal appears to be the autistic child's perceptual repertoire. A limited set of stimuli control his behavior, and an increase in stimulus complexity disrupts this control.

Ferster proposes that all of these characteristics of autistic children can be viewed as having developed as the result of their reinforcement history, that is, the circumstances in the early life of these children. If the difference between the autistic child and the normal child is in the frequency with which given behavior occurs, a functional analysis will ask how the response frequency is affected by the effect responses have on the environment. The answer is that when behavior is not reinforced or is reinforced only intermittently, it will be emitted at low frequency, may fail to develop, or may become extinguished. This would be the case where parents fail to respond to the child or do so on an erratic schedule. Ferster speculates that parents who are preoccupied with behavior that is prepotent over caretaking activities or whose own repertoire is disrupted by somatic disturbances, diseases, or depression are parents who find dealing with a child aversive and less rewarding than alternative activities.

When parents fail to respond to a child's behavior when it is emitted at low magnitude, it may undergo extinction; but when they then selectively attend to such high magnitude responses as tantrums, these come to be strengthened, resulting in the relatively low frequency of social behaviors and in the relatively high frequency of atavisms. At the same time, a child who finds his parents only occasionally presenting him with reinforcing stimuli will discover that his behavior has a consistent and predictable effect on the nonsocial, physical environment. The doorknob at the end of a string exerts a mild pull whenever the string is jerked, and while this pulling effect is a weak reinforcing stimulus, its durability and ready availability in the face of the absence of stronger, social reinforcers comes to maintain the string-jerking behavior. Furthermore, the parent is not likely to interfere with such noiseless, nonirritating behavior while he may actively discourage behavior that would have a greater effect on the environment, such as handling household objects, playing with toys, or moving objects about the house. This, Ferster believes, accounts for the fact that a large part of the autistic child's repertoire consists of behaviors that have small, limited effects on the physical environment. By similar reasoning, he explains that the child's failure to acquire conditioned and generalized reinforcers for his reduced overall performance is seen as interfering with the development and effectiveness of such reinforcers.

The limited number of stimuli that control the autistic child's behavior is, according to Ferster's formulations, the result of the narrow range of conditions under which the child's behavior is reinforced. Where this is the case, behavior would not be emitted under conditions that are dissimilar from those under which it was learned, and sudden shifts in stimuli are likely to elicit emotional responses that may interfere with established performance. Ferster cites a case where a child's behavior became disrupted when a previously constant companion, a babysitter, suddenly departed.

Ferster concludes his hypothetical analysis of the development of infantile autism by stressing the cumulative effects of behavioral deficits. During the first four years of a child's life, his parents can have such exclusive control over the conditions reinforcing the child's behavior that their atypical contingency management could produce the gross behavioral deficits seen in the autistic child. Once such a child becomes exposed to the larger community after age four, he is unlikely to develop a normal behavioral repertoire because the community tends to reinforce only age-appropriate behavior. To make it possible for a parent to have exclusive control over a child's contingencies of reinforcement, Ferster has to postulate that the child's environment contains a limited number of such people as siblings, relatives, and neighbors, who might attenuate the social isolation where one parent can be the sole source of reinforcement. Accordingly, he expects that severely disturbed autistic children are, in general, firstborn children raised in physically or socially isolated families.

While available data (Wing, 1966) support the speculation that the majority (54 percent) of autistic children are firstborn, we have no information to support the contention that autistic children come from isolated homes or from families where one parent is largely absent. Nor does the available literature provide support for the presence of the postulated parental characteristics which call for general disruption of the parental behavior repertoire and a prepotency of other than child-caring performances, resulting in a large amount of intermittent reinforcement of the child's day-to-day behavior. It must, furthermore, be recalled that children reared in understimulating, overcrowded institutions where behavior is likely to be reinforced on highly erratic, intermittent schedules have never been reported as developing early infantile autism, although they do display limited behavior repertoires and cognitive defects. Pending the accumulation of the kind of objective assessment and direct observations called for in Ferster's provocative paper, his formulations must be considered no more than challenging hypotheses that would, if confirmed, make parental behavior the sole factor causing the development of early infantile autism.

Ferster's operant formulations, derived from Skinner's (1953) view of human behavior, bear a remarkable similarity to the theorizing of such traditional psychoanalysts as Bettelheim (1967) in that both view infantile autism as primarily the result of parental behavior. Bettelheim views the parental environment as responsible for the fact that the child is not exposed to experiences that are vital for his normal development. While Bettelheim invokes unconscious maternal wishes that the child did not exist and Ferster prefers to make no such motivational assumptions, both formulations lead to the conclusion that the parents are to blame for the fact that their child is autistic.

The parents of autistic children are often described as of better than average, frequently superior intelligence. There is said to be a high incidence of professionals with graduate degrees among them. They are frequently pictured as "emotionally cold," introspective, detached, and excessively objective. Their child-rearing practices are said to be characterized by a "mechanization" of parent-child relations. Rimland (1964) searched the available literature for support for these descriptions and found that the picture of the cold, reserved, efficient, and highly intelligent parent was presented in most reports. While the descriptions of these parents tend to be consistent in many cases, one must not lose sight of the fact that these parental characteristics may be an artifact, especially since more careful assessment fails to confirm the hypothesis that parents of autistic children are intellectually brilliant and emotionally cold (Wolff & Morris, 1971). None of these parents are ever seen until *after* their child has been diagnosed as autistic, and by that time they have usually been living with the grossly atypical behavior of this child for several years. At that point, it is not surprising that they are found to be "disdainful of frivolity, humorless" (Rimland, 1964, p. 25) and that the interaction with their child is remarkably different from the expected norm. A study by Klebanoff (1959) strongly suggests that having a seriously disturbed child affects maternal attitudes to childrearing and that a formulation that views these attitudes as contributing to the child's disturbance may be reversing the causal sequence.

Any theoretical speculation about the basis of early infantile autism that seeks to find causation in the parental characteristics described must also deal with the following facts: where autistic children have siblings, these are almost invariably described as normal; autistic characteristics are present from the time of birth; and the sex ratio among autistic children is of the order of 3 or 4 boys to 1 girl. Finally, there is the fact that when sets of twins are autistic, these are almost invariably identical pairs. Rimland (1964), who reviewed all 200 or so "bonafide cases of autism referred to in the literature," (p. 57) identified eleven monozygotic twins— concordant for infantile autism.

Cognitive Defect

At the pole opposite the environmentalist position of such theorists as Bettelheim and Ferster stands the neurophysiological speculation of Rimland (1964). That writer concluded from a thorough review of the available literature that infantile autism can be traced to one single critical deficiency in the child's cognitive function—an impaired ability to relate new stimuli to remembered experience. A child with such an impairment would be severely limited in deriving benefit from his experience, each event being, as it were, totally new and without relation to anything that transpired in the past. As a result, the child would be unable to understand relationships or to think in terms of such abstractions as symbols, concepts, and analogies. Unable to integrate his sensations into a comprehensible whole, he would perceive the world as vague, obscure, overwhelming, and frightening. Since there would be little or no carry-over of an experience with a given individual from one occasion to the next, people would fail to acquire meaning, and interpersonal relationships would be impossible.

The postulated basic deficit in relating perceptions to memory would also explain the language difficulties of autistic children and why many of them do no more than parrot words they have just heard, a phenomenon called *echolalia*. The characteristic insistence on sameness—near panic when even minor changes are made in their surroundings—and stereotyped preoccupation with inanimate objects can be viewed as attempts on the part of these children to minimize the confusing effects of their deficit. It is likely that even with their impairment, stimuli that are presented in identical fashion time and time again will eventually come to be associated with their consequences so that change or removal of these stimuli elicits an emotional response.

In addition to postulating the cognitive defect that might mediate the behavior of autistic children, Rimland (1964) speculates on the nature of the physiological basis of this defect. He suggests that the reticular formation of the brainstem is the structure whose integrity is crucial for the integration of memory with current perceptions and assumes that damage to this structure manifests itself in the impairment shown by autistic children. On the basis of his reading of the available literature, Rimland further suggests that an excess of oxygen during early infancy might be responsible for the reticular damage. Since there are great individual differences in reactivity to oxygen, even the oxygen level naturally available in the atmosphere might exceed the tolerance level of some genetically predisposed infants.

The hypotheses advanced by Rimland, though plausible on the basis of available knowledge, require careful scientific investigation before they can be viewed as correct explanations for the development and nature of early infantile autism. The theory has the merit of accounting for the available facts, listed earlier, and it has the advantage of not placing blame for the condition on the behavior of the child's parents. Considering the tenuous basis and lack of scientific support for the assumption that the mother's personality is somehow to blame, it is pernicious to compound the tremendous difficulties a mother has in trying to raise a child who is autistic by burdening her with the undocumented and unconstructive guilt that further complicates her relationship to her child.

Stimulus Overselectivity

A formulation of infantile autism in terms of the child's inability to respond adaptively when several stimuli are presented simultaneously has been advanced by Lovaas, Schreibman, Koegel and Rehm (1971). While these authors do not relate their formulation to the speculations of Rimland (1964), it is possible to conceive of "remembered experience" as stimuli which are presented simultaneously with present events so that together they represent a stimulus complex to which the child is unable to respond. At any rate, Lovaas et al. (1971) base their formulation on experimental data which have a bearing on the problem no matter how one wishes to interpret them. Five autistic children ranging in age from four to ten years (mean = 7.2 years), five mentally retarded children (mean MA = 3.7), and five normal children with a mean chronological age of 6.4 were trained to respond with a bar press to a stimulus complex consisting of simultaneously presented auditory, visual, and tactile cues. Once the child had learned to discriminate the stimulus complex, the investigators examined which of the stimuli within the complex controlled the response by introducing test trials on which only one of the three stimuli was presented.

The results showed that the autistic children responded primarily to only one of the cues while the normals responded uniformly to all three. The retarded group functioned between these two extremes. It was also shown that the problem of the autistic children was not that they were impaired in one or another sense modality but that, when presented with a stimulus complex, their responding showed, what the authors call, *stimulus over-selectivity.* Instead of attending to the complex, the autistic children seemed to attend, or be able to attend, to only one aspect of the complex.

If one recognizes that learning involves the contiguous or near-contiguous pairing of two or more stimuli, failure to respond to one of these stimuli can be viewed as an important factor in the development of the difficulties manifested by the autistic child. As Lovaas and his colleagues (1971) point out, the acquisition of interpersonal and intellectual behavior is based on the prior acquisition of conditioned reinforcers, which involves their contiguous association with primary reinforcers. Furthermore, the establishment of appropriate affect may involve the contiguous presentation of two stimulus events so that the affect elicited by one of these events (the UCS) can come to be elicited by the other (the CS). Language acquisition, in terms of learning the meaning of words, again involves pairing of stimuli, as does the acquisition of new behavioral topographies. If a child were to attend to only one of a complex of contiguously presented stimuli, a grossly impoverished behavioral repertoire, so typical of the autistic child, might be the expected outcome. Further research along this line may well contribute to an unravelling of the complex phenomenon that is called *early infantile autism*.

Sensory and Affective Defect

In Rimland's formulation, early infantile autism stems from a basic cognitive defect, the inability to relate present sensory stimuli to past experience. This would explain the phenomenon of autistic aloneness on the basis that the child is unable to acquire interpersonal attachments because the stimulus constellation represented by his mother and other persons fails to become associated with pleasurable experiences. This, in turn, would explain the absence of the social smile (of recognition), anticipatory movements to being picked up, and the failure to enjoy simple interpersonal games. Failure in the development of such affective components of behavior as pleasure is thus seen as secondary to failure in the development of necessary associations. When Kanner (1943) first described autistic disturbances, he emphasized the affective component as central to the problem and, in fact, referred to it as an inborn affective disturbance. The issue whether infantile autism is an associational deficit *or* an affective deficit is resolved in a formulation presented by

DesLauriers and Carlson (1969) who reason that sensory *and* affective processes might be defective in the case of children in the category early infantile autism.

DesLauriers and Carlson emphasize that the learning necessary for human development requires attending not only to stimulation but also to the association between stimulation, responses, and rewards. They propose that on a neurophysiological level, two arousal systems must operate in order for perception, attention, motivation, learning, and affect to take place in a normal adaptive fashion. Arousal System I, presumably located in the brainstem reticular formation, is postulated as serving as the source of activation and energy, while Arousal System II, thought to be found in the limbic-midbrain system, is seen as mediating incentive, reward, and positive reinforcement functions. These two arousal systems are said to operate in a reciprocal fashion and to require balance for optimal adaptation. Figure 5 depicts the relationship of these arousal systems as postulated for a well-functioning individual. Both systems operate within the normal activity level (vertical axis);

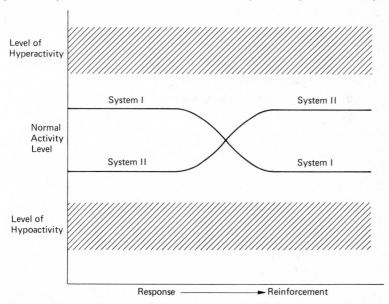

Fig. 5. The relationship of the two arousal systems as postulated by DesLauriers and Carlson. (Redrawn from DesLauriers and Carlson, 1969.)

when a response is emitted, System I is ascendant, but when re-inforcement takes place, ascendancy is reversed with System II temporarily becoming predominant. Various deviations from normal functioning can be expected if the two systems operate at either too high or too low a level of activity, if they are not in equilibrium, or if the reversal of ascendancy fails to take place.

DesLauriers and Carlson describe the deficiency of the autistic child in these terms :

> The imbalance is in the direction of sustained ascendency of System I over System II; i.e., sustained suppression or inhibition of System II by System I. The result of this purported imbalance is a severe disturbance of affect; severe limitation of learning, or ability to establish meaningful associations; and goalless, aimless, repetitive, and stereotyped behavior, without any apparent adaptive value aside from pure stimulus input [1969, p. 64].

DesLauriers and Carlson thus speculate that in the autistic child, arousal is primarily a function of the activation-drive-energy system. This would mean that the child, though able to attend to new stimuli and to emit responses, would be severely handicapped in associating responses and rewards, since System II would not function adequately in suppressing System I long enough for such association to take place. As a result, most incoming stimuli would be perceived as new and unfamiliar.

The model offers a mode of conceptualizing the phenomena of autistic aloneness (in that the child lacks the capacity to experience affect) and preservation of sameness (since stereotyped behavior is the only behavior the child can learn). Since the dysfunction of the two arousal systems is seen as an inborn organic deficiency, it follows that the child's parents cannot be blamed for their child's autistic condition. The end product of this neurophysiological model is thus similar to the impairment postulated by Rimland, except that the two-arousal system theory also accounts for affective impairments if one attributes the "pleasure" associated with reward to System II, as DesLauriers and Carlson suggest.

There are two circumstances under which autistic children seem to display learning. One is when there has been an exceedingly long series of repetitious presentations of discriminative and reinforcing stimuli (as in stereotyped routines or operant conditioning trials), the other when a training trial is presented under conditions of unusually strong affective arousal. The DesLauriers and Carlson model accounts for these instances by postulating that these circumstances force momentary ascendance of System II.

DesLauriers and Carlson use their neurophysiological model to support a treatment approach with which they report remarkable success with a small number of children. Since all children with early infantile autism are viewed as incapable of being aroused by the levels of affective stimulation existing in the normal environment, a therapist must, in order to overcome this "affective barrier," expose these children to "high-impact, affective stimulation of a consistent, persistent, and well-structured nature" (p. 67). Since these authors further differentiate between the hyperactive, hypersensitive and the hypoactive, hyposensitive autistic child, they further go on to say that the latter child must not only be "bombarded with high affective stimulation, but [that] all other types of stimulation . . . primarily tactile, proprioceptive, and kinesthetic, which serve as the vehicles of the affective stimulation must *also* be of high impact—either by virtue of initial strength or excessive repetition" (ibid.). The hyperactive, hypersensitive autistic child, on the other hand, should not have tactile, proprioceptive, and kinesthetic stimulation exceeding the normal levels, although he too must be exposed to high-impact affective stimulation.

The emphasis on near-receptors (those involving direct contact with the body) as opposed to distance receptors (sight, hearing, and smell) derives from the conviction of DesLauriers and Carlson that the developmentally and phylogenetically more primitive near-receptors play a vital role in helping the child differentiate and separate himself as an individual—to form what they call a "body image" which they describe "as the sum total of physical, sensory contacts between the child and the mother" and view as "the instrument of relationship and communication between these two" (pp. 13f.). For normal development to take place, there has to be a bodily interaction between mother and infant, with the infant seeking stimulation and the parent responding. These authors suggest that infantile autism develops because the child "not only does not reach out for human contacts, he is also unreachable by those around him who try to contact him" (p. 15). The autistic child does not take the initiative in seeking stimulation which he must if adequate parental responding is to be elicited. Not only does the parent have no response to give "but the incentive to give a response progressively dies, and the parent eventually appears just as distant from the child as the child is from the parent" (p. 15). This formulation is similar to that of *attachment defect,* to be discussed in the next section.

In their emphasis on near-receptors, DesLauriers and Carlson are in agreement with a hypothesis advanced by Schopler (1965) who was also led to recommend a form of treatment aimed at stimulating near-receptors through bodily contact. One of the most salutary consequences of this formulation is that treatment becomes not an arcane ritual performed in the secrecy of the playroom but an educational process in which the child's family and teachers are urged to participate. They are instructed to provide highly impactful, affective stimulation and to offer the child a wide variety of sensory experiences through tactile, kinesthetic, and proprioceptive contacts. Parents are encouraged to engage in the same playful interactions they would with a normal child except that they are to do so more forcefully, more playfully, more persistently, "just more of everything" (p. 171). At the same time as this playful, joyful interaction is forced upon the child in a highly intrusive manner, the adult is expected to impose controls on the child's behavior; preventing disorganized, purposeless, and aimless activity.

As pointed out, DesLauriers and Carlson report remarkable success with the five young children whom they treated in this manner. To what extent their success is a function of their ability "to be spontaneously capable of genuinely playful activity with the child" (p. 138) and to what extent the approach can be taught to others remains to be seen. It is difficult to share their satisfaction when they write, "Fortunately, our approach could not be encompassed by a recipe book of specific techniques; rather it emphasized an attitude toward the child, a climate in which the child came alive, a structure that enhanced the conditions of growth in the child" (p. 171). A therapeutic approach does not have to be reduced to a cookbook to be teachable, but unless attitude and climate can be operationalized, others may find it difficult to benefit from the work of DesLauriers and Carlson.

The difficulty in communicating what is meant by "affective climate" in such a way that others can reproduce the treatment conditions employed by DesLauriers and Carlson is particularly unfortunate since their method seems so successful. Each of the children in the project was given repeated tests by someone other than the therapists before, during, and at termination of treatment. These tests included the Vineland Social Maturity Scale, selected parts of the Fels Behavior Scales, and age-appropriate tests of intelligence. Of the five original children in the project, the four children who remained for at least 1 year showed highly significant changes in their test pattern on the Fels scales, reflecting improvement in such areas as curiosity, playfulness, and obedience. On the Vineland scale they showed equally significant improvement (beyond the 0.001 level of confidence) in such skills as communication, self-help, socialization, and language. Inasmuch as language deficit is probably the most crucial from the point of view of the social adaptation of the autistic child and since a child who has failed to develop language by age five has generally been viewed as having very poor prognosis (Eisenberg, 1956), it is of particular interest to examine in some detail the changes in language reported for the children treated in the DesLauriers project.

The child identified as Kathy, who began treatment when she was 2 years, 9 months old, was described as initially mute and without receptive language. At the end of treatment, 26 months later, she was reported as having "full receptive language" with expressive language developing normally and at a rapid rate. Elizabeth, who was 3 years, 3 months old when treatment began, made the same progress in a 14-month treatment period. Tommy, age 2 years, 3 months at onset of treatment, had neither receptive nor expressive language initially and 14 months later was described as having good receptive but little expressive language. June, who was 4 years, 10 months at onset of treatment, initially displayed receptive language selectively and "immature expressive language with some autistic-like peculiarities." At the end of treatment, 13 months later, she was reported as having "full receptive language and wide expressive language without autistic characteristics." A girl identified as Connie was the oldest child in the group. When treatment began, she was 5 years, 1 month of age and had neither receptive nor expressive language. When she was abruptly taken out of treatment 11 months later, there was little improvement in expressive but definite improvement in receptive language.

While the number of children is too small for meaningful generalization, the progress they made would seem to support the expectation that the younger the child when treatment is initiated, the better his chances of developing normal language. The older the child at onset of treatment, the longer the period during which autistic behavior has been reinforced, the more opportunities for learning adaptive behavior have been missed, and the greater the degree of parental despair. DesLauriers and Carlson look to this last point, parental feelings of hopelessness, for an explanation of the relative treatment failure with Connie and her abrupt termination. They point out that three treatment sessions per week on an out-patient basis cannot possibly lead to success unless the parents are able to maintain the child at home on the same high-impact affective stimulation which is the basis of treatment at the clinic. A treatment approach that counts on parental participation has no chance of success where parents are unable to cooperate. The implication of this would seem to be that therapists must attempt to modify the behavior of parents at the same time, or even before they attempt treatment with the child. Not all parents can be expected to be successful cotherapists with as little effort as DesLauriers and Carlson apparently extended in that direction.

Attachment Defect

A formulation about the development of early infantile autism that bears a certain similarity to that advanced by DesLauriers and Carlson is one offered by Zaslow and Breger (1969). Extrapolating from the observations of ethologists and other students of the early development of nonhuman species, these authors point out that an essential step in social development is the formation of the infant's attachment to his mother. They postulate that this formation of attachment does not take place in the case of the autistic child. Attachment, they suggest, is a function of the early infant-mother interaction to which the infant contributes as much as the mother. Autistic children, they speculate, are less "cuddly" than the average baby, the quality of "cuddlyness" presumably being a normally distributed, constitutional trait. When an infant who is low in "cuddlyness" happens to have a mother who redoubles her efforts at physical contact with him, his development may well be un-remarkable. On the other hand, when the mother reacts to this constitutional quality of her child by reducing her physical contact with him—thus depriving him of the kinesthetic, tactual, visual, and auditory stimuli associated with being held—the child will be unable to form the crucial attachment which, in part, derives from being held while passing through periods of stress and rage.

This theoretical speculation of Zaslow and Breger thus points to a *mismatch* between infant and mother as the source of infantile autism. The child is low in "cuddlyness," and the mother reduces her contact with him; he, in turn, is deprived of the stimuli associated with being held which are particularly crucial for the formation of attachment during episodes of intense arousal. The failure to form attachment then leads to the characteristic autistic phenomena. The child will not learn the social smile, will fail to acquire language, and will be unable to relate to the social environment. Instead, humans will be actively avoided, and the child will attempt to master the nonhuman environment on his own terms. This formulation would thus account for the three foremost characteristics of the autistic child: absence of language, autistic aloneness, and preservation of sameness.

Their emphasis on the importance of being physically held during periods of rage and stress leads Zaslow and Breger to a therapeutic approach, the "rage reduction method," which emphasizes holding of the child in close body contact until rage episodes subside. They view it as essential that the therapist establish the fact that he is "in charge," thus interrupting the child's negativistic response system which centers around self-initiated, self-maintained actions. While this form of treatment is reported to work for some children, its long-range effectiveness has not yet been demonstrated; and even if it had, the effectiveness of treatment would not be a test of the validity of the rather loose causal speculations. This formulation was included in the discussion because in its emphasis on the interaction between constitution and environment and the transaction between infant and mother, it represents a logical link in the chain of causal theories that range from Rimland's genetic-neurophysiological model to Ferster's radical environmentalism.

Defective Arousal Mechanism

It is of interest that DesLauriers and Carlson (1969) and Zaslow and Breger (1969) independently but simultaneously and by rather different theoretical routes arrived at treatment approaches that have a great deal in common. Both emphasize stimulation of the near receptors, both stress the importance of high levels of stimulation (rage in one case, intense pleasure in the other), and both would have the therapist forcefully intrude in the child's autistic world and disrupt his stereotyped perseverations. If, as both sets of authors report, their treatment is effective, one would need to look to these common elements for hypotheses about the defects involved in early infantile autism.

Intrusive insistence on tactile, kinesthetic, and proprioceptive stimulation under conditions of high affective excitation appear to be the common ingredients of the therapies devised by Schopler (1962), Zaslow and Breger (1969), and DesLauriers and Carlson (1969). Near receptors are developmentally more primitive; their development precedes that of the distance receptors both phylogenetically and ontogenetically. If the autistic child can be stimulated more effectively via near receptors, it might mean that treatment must attempt to recapitulate certain aspects of the child's development—aspects that were ineffective in establishing the child's responsiveness to his environment because of his high-stimulus threshold. It is such a high threshold which would demand that stimulation be insistently intrusive and that it be brought to bear while the child is in a high state of excitation, as is the case in rage or intense pleasure.

Several writers see the need to expose the autistic child to high levels of stimulation as related to the child's arousal level. The construct *arousal* is, like many such constructs, rather vaguely defined. As used by Berlyne (1960), arousal motivates behavior in that the organism seeks to maintain his arousal at an optimal level. When arousal is below this optimal level, as in a state of boredom, the organism will seek to increase stimulation and, hence, arousal; when arousal is above the optimal level, as in high excitement, the organism will seek to reduce stimulation and, with it, arousal. It is further thought that learning is facilitated by high arousal although extreme arousal disrupts the acquisition of new responses. If what is "optimal" varies from individual to individual, it would explain why some students of autistic children (e.g., Metz, 1967) report that these children seek higher-than-normal levels of stimulation while others (e.g., Hutt, et al., 1965) find that they are in a chronically high state of physiological arousal.

If one assumes that autistic children have a defective arousal system, it would suggest that many of them would require high-intensity stimulation for effective learning while for others this would not be necessary. DesLauriers and Carlson recognized this when they differentiated between the hyposensitive and the hypersensitive autistic child. A study by Metz (1967) lends strong support to the assumption that some autistic children require a higher intensity of stimulation for effective learning than do normal children. He compared ten autistic, ten schizophrenic, and ten "outstandingly successful" children in a situation where they were able to control the volume of tape-recorded sound by operating a lever. The autistic children selected significantly higher volume settings than the normal, while the schizophrenic children were more variable in their choice of settings.

It has been suggested that some of the atavistic, at times self-injurious behavior, such as rocking and head banging, represent a similar "turning up of input volume" on the part of the autistic child at a chronically low level of arousal whose behavior is reinforced by the resulting high stimulation. While we know of no study, analogous to that of Metz, that demonstrates stimulus-reducing behavior on the part of autistic children, recollections about the early infancy of autistic children often include reports of the infant arching his body away from his mother when she tried to hold him. This may represent the infant's avoidance responses to stimuli that are, to him, of too high an intensity, and thus aversive. Similarly, the frequent descriptions of autistic children who walk around covering their ears with their hands may tell of children trying to reduce stimulation to which they are hypersensitive.

Whether one wishes to adduce a motivational construct like arousal in order to explain human behavior is largely a matter of theoretical preference. Arousal has the advantage in that it has demonstrable physiological correlates, it enables one to order a number of discrete empirical facts, and it serves to generate testable hypotheses. It thus meets the requirements of a good theory and deserves consideration.

RESEARCH

Research that might throw light on the nature of early infantile autism is made difficult not only by the classificatory confusion to which we have already alluded but also by the low incidence of this disorder which limits the number of children any one investigator might study even in a lifetime devoted to research. As a result, studies purporting to deal with early infantile autism often include children who do not meet the restricting criteria proposed by Rimland (1964), for example, those with obvious neurological disorders. Thus, Ritvo, Ornitz, and LaFranchi (1968), in a study of the repetitive behaviors in "early infantile autism and its variants," included among their fifteen subjects a child with chronic brain disease associated with phenylketonuria that had not been diagnosed until he was $4\frac{1}{2}$ years old. What all the children did have in common, in addition to the somewhat questionable diagnosis of early infantile autism, was a long history of repetitive behaviors.

The Ritvo, Ornitz, and LaFranchi research showed that repetitive behaviors are not reactions to the environment but that they are initiated and maintained by involuntary processes in the central nervous system. This conclusion was based on analyses of motion pictures of the typically repetitive flapping, clapping, oscillating, and rocking movements of these children. The data showed stable response rate from the beginning to the end of the episode. There was no speedup or slowdown in relation to changes in the child's presumed emotional state, as judged from his overt appearance. For all but body rocking, high consistency in rate was also noted when a given child's behavior was compared from one episode to the next and when comparisons between the rates of different children were made. One might assume that the variability in response rate within and between children would be far greater if, as some writers have held, the repetitive behavior were the symbolic representation of the child's hallucinatory fantasy. The authors of this study suggest that it is more likely that the behavior is involuntary and the result of a dysfunction of the central nervous system, possibly an imbalance between the excitatory and inhibitory control of motor responses.

Another study in which autistic children were mixed with other psychotic children was one reported by Hagen, Winsberg, and Wolff (1968). This work also illustrates the conceptual confusion that plagues this area of inquiry. It will be recalled that Rimland suggested that defective memory function precludes adequate language development. Hagen and his colleagues, on the other hand, reason that language is vital to such functions as memory for immediate past experience. They therefore compared the performance of ten psychotic children at various levels of language functioning with a group of normal controls. All but two of the psychotic children were described as autistic or with "autistic features," but several of them had demonstrable central nervous system damage. The children were tested on tasks requiring discrimination, transposition, generalization, reversal shift, and short-term memory with and without verbal cues. As expected, the psychotic children performed worse than the normals on all tasks, and language ability was directly related to the adequacy of performance on memory and discrimination learning tasks.

This study highlights the central role that deficient language plays in the behavioral difficulties of autistic children. A child who fails to develop language for whatever reason is obviously under a gross handicap. The question whether language deficit is the cause or the effect of the cognitive difficulties of autistic children is, of course, not answered by the Hagen, Winsberg, and Wolff study. All it shows is that language impairment is correlated with other cognitive defects. To test the causal hypothesis, one would need to teach language to a nonverbal child under carefully controlled conditions and then assess whether this produces improvement in his discriminative ability and memory. Such a study remains to be done.

Viewing language disorder as the dominant problem of autistic children, Frith (1970) noted the paradox that these children fail to perceive structure yet appear preoccupied with structure. They will, for example, fail to respond to the content of a verbal message yet perseverate in repeating this message over and over again. Frith proposed that this paradox can be understood by postulating an imbalance between "feature extraction" and "pattern imposition." According to this hypothesis, the inability to perceive meaning would be explained by failure of feature extraction, while the tendency to stereotyped behavior would be accounted for by a dominance of pattern imposition. To demonstrate the operation of this deficit in feature extraction, Frith conducted a study comparing immediate recall of binary verbal sequences of autistic, normal, and subnormal children. The children were asked to reproduce verbal sequences of two types. One type involved a cyclic pattern (*ababab*), as in "come here come here come here"; the other a noncyclic pattern (*abbbaa*), as in "lets go go go lets lets." The results of the study were in line with the hypothesis in that the autistic children had little difficulty recalling quasi-random material but were impaired in processing meaningful material. While the normal, and to some extent the subnormal children were able to rely on the appropriate rule—depending on whether the sequence contained predominantly alternating or repeating elements—the autistic children would reconstruct the lists on the basis of a perseveration rule, regardless of whether or not redundancy was the predominant feature of the list. In terms of the hypothesis, the control group showed feature extraction, while the autistic subjects showed evidence of pattern imposition, independent of input.

This work would seem to confirm the frequent observation that autistic children are unable to extract meaning from verbal messages. While the results are in line with the postulated "imbalance between two mechanisms," the existence of such mechanisms is in no way confirmed and to say that the autistic children "applied a rule" goes considerably beyond the data. As Frith (1970) points out, it remains to be seen whether autistic children always respond in terms of perseveration "or whether another type of structure would be preferred in other conditions" (p. 419).

The failure of the autistic child to respond to simple commands and requests and the difficulty with which he learns to perform simple responses have, at times, been ascribed to *negativism*—a motivation not to emit a requested response. This hypothesis was investigated by Cowan, Hoddinott, and Wright (1965) who studied the behavior of twelve children between the ages of 4 and 9 who had been carefully selected to meet the restricted definition of early infantile autism. The children were individually trained to pick up skeins of colored wool and deposit them in a box. The behavior was modeled by the examiner and reinforced with pieces of popcorn. After this response had been established, the child was given verbal instructions to place a specified object into the box. The objects were small colored tiles in the shapes of circles, squares, and triangles; and the requests were either for a square or for a red tile. The multiple-choice procedure used made it possible to compare the number of correct choices made by each child with the number of correct choices possible by chance. Only two of the twelve subjects obtained perfect scores; all others made *fewer* correct choices than chance would allow. That is, they were wrong more often than they would have been had they picked up the objects with their eyes closed. Since the correct choice was thus studiously avoided, it seemed clear that the children must have understood the request and known which object was the correct one. The authors conclude somewhat precipitately that "negativism, rather than indifference, lack of capacity, or lack of experience, is the only possible way of accounting for the failure of the ten *S*s to give correct responses" (p. 919).

In the first part of the experiment just described, every response, regardless of correctness, had been rewarded "in order to keep *S* interested in the task" (Cowan, et al., 1965, p. 916). Other than the experimenter's request, "Put a red one in the box," the condition thus did not contain any cues as to the correctness of the child's response. With red, blue, yellow, and green tiles of various shapes before him, the child was presented with the above request. Regardless of the tile picked up, he would receive a reward. This means that if he picked up a blue tile on the first trial, he was reinforced for *not* following the experimenter's instructions. Reinforcement theory would predict that on the next trial he should pick up the same blue tile, but the test conditions prevented this because the tile picked up on the immediately preceding trial was withheld during the next trial in order to prevent *S*s "from perseverative responding" (ibid.). With the response that had just been reinforced thus prevented from being emitted, the child may well have learned a response class, that is, *not* following instructions. The fact that group data showed a decline in the number of correct choices in each succeeding block of five trials adds plausibility to this explanation. What is demonstrated then need not be called *motivational negativism*; it may simply be learning of a reinforced response class.

The second part of the Cowan et al. experiment seems to lend further support to the interpretation just advanced. The purpose was to test whether "the negativism could be overcome when the incentive conditions were changed" (p. 920). Instructions and task remained the same, but reinforcement was given *only* when the child emitted a correct response. Working only with the children who had given significantly few correct responses in the earlier sessions, five were now trained to present red tiles and five to present square tiles. Two days later, all children were retested on both the "red" and the "square" trials from the first part of the study. With this procedure, four of the ten subjects learned to make nothing but correct responses on both kinds of posttests. That is, those who had been trained on squares presented not only squares but also red appropriately. They had learned to follow the experimenter's instructions because following instructions had been reinforced during training trials. To say that the procedure had "overcome the negativistic behavior" (p. 921) seems to invoke an unnecessary construct. As for the six children who failed to learn to follow instructions, it is quite possible that, as Cowan et al. themselves suggest, different or larger rewards might have been more effective in establishing compliant responses.

Cowan et al. pointed out that the two children who gave correct responses throughout the first part of the experiment were the only two in the sample who used some language. These, plus five of the six who learned the compliance response in the second part of the study, also had the highest intelligence test scores. All six compliers are also reported to have succeeded on a concept learning task—which the six noncompliers had failed—and, in yet another study, compliers seemed to learn cooperative behavior more readily than non-compliers. All of this seems to suggest consistent differences in learning ability rather than resistance or negativism.

OPERANT CONDITIONING

Investigators who study early infantile autism from the operant frame of reference approach their problem not by asking, "What is wrong with the autistic child?" as did the writers whose work was discussed thus far, but by observing a behavior deficit and asking, "How can I teach the child to overcome this deficit?"

One of the deficits frequently reported as typical of autistic children is their failure to imitate other people. In operant terminology: other people do not serve as discriminative stimuli that might control the behavior of autistic children. Since the discriminative characteristic of a stimulus has to be learned, this would be another instance of the autistic child's failure to learn a "tool" response—the lack of which, in turn, prevents him from acquiring other response patterns through modeling (Bandura, 1969). In a study reported in 1965, Metz used operant conditioning methods to teach two autistic children to imitate simple behaviors of an adult. The children, a boy and a girl, both seven years old, had been hospitalized for 1 and $2\frac{1}{2}$ years, respectively, and had shown little, if any, response to conventional therapeutic programs. Working with them at lunchtime on days when they had not been given breakfast, Metz used food, tokens that could be traded for food, and the word "good" to reinforce imitative behavior and to establish generalized imitation.

To qualify as generalized imitation, a response must meet the following conditions: It must be topographically similar to the response demonstrated by the model; it must be emitted on the occasion of the specific example shown by the model; the model's behavior must serve as discriminative stimulus for the subject who must respond differentially to different responses by the model; and the behavior being imitated must be relatively novel as an item under the control of the model's exemplar; that is, it must be an item that the child has not been specifically taught to perform in response to the model's presentation.

Metz used such items as kicking a beanbag, putting a blanket on a doll, riding a hobby horse, placing a block into a box, and blowing a whistle. Working with each child individually, Metz used one list of such items to pretest for imitative behavior. At this point, the boy emitted five imitative responses, the girl none. The children were then taught a repertoire of six tasks, using passive demonstration and shaping procedures, with correct responses followed by the delivery of reinforcement. A task was considered learned when it was correctly performed six times in a row when presented in a series with the five other tasks. To reach this criterion, the boy required ten sessions and the girl five; the sessions were one-half to three-quarters of an hour in length. The six learned tasks were next interspersed with fourteen new tasks. Ten of these were reinforced when correctly imitated; four were nonrewarded tasks which were included to test for extinction. A task was considered imitated when it had been correctly performed on two out of three trials. This phase of the study was followed by further, more intensive training on additional items, further testing for generalization, and finally a post-testing with an entirely new list. On that occasion, the boy made eleven, the girl thirteen correct, imitative responses out of a possible total of sixteen. Generalized imitation had thus increased for both children although, without a control, it is not entirely certain that this increase was the result of the training procedures employed. One must nonetheless concur with Metz that the results suggest that autistic children can learn to imitate, that such learning can generalize to similar but new behaviors without specific training, and that the generalized imitative response can persist—in the context of reinforcement of *other* imitative behavior—without specifically being reinforced (p. 397).

Therapists using operant procedures to teach autistic children are frequently accused of ignoring the affective element of the child's behavior, particularly by those who, like DesLauriers and Carlson

(1969), place heavy emphasis on affective aspects in their own therapeutic efforts. In this light, the following subjective observations, reported by Metz, are of particular interest:

> ... as appropriate learning occurred, "inappropriate" motor and emotional behavior spontaneously disappeared. Not only did the children learn to do what was required by the task, but appropriate emotional responses also seemed to appear. For example, the children expressed joy or delight upon "solving" a problem, an affect rarely seen in these children in other situations. The children eventually appeared to enjoy the whole procedure, sought *E* out whenever he appeared on the ward, ran eagerly to the experimental room, etc. [Metz, 1965, p. 398].

While operant methods do not specifically deal with joy and delight, it seems that when these methods succeed in teaching a child adaptive responses that lead to positive reinforcement, positive affect appears spontaneously, as if the child enjoyed his newfound competence.

One highly effective approach to teaching autistic children certain adaptive behaviors is found in the work of Lovaas and his coworkers (e.g., Lovaas, Freitas, Nelson, & Whalen, 1967). Lovaas places almost exclusive emphasis on the use of operant methods in gradually building a behavior repertoire in the children seen in his laboratory. This means that discrete stimuli are repeated over and over again until the desired response is clearly established through immediate, initially continuous reinforcement. In one of his earlier reports Lovaas (1966) spoke of a program used to establish speech which involved training sessions lasting from 2 to 7 hours per day. During the training sessions, the child and his teacher sit with their heads about one foot apart and, when necessary, "the adult physically prevented the child from leaving the situation by holding the child's legs between his own legs" (p. 123). It would thus seem that the method not only is insistingly intrusive in terms of the massing of trials but also contains some physical contact and thus near-receptor stimulation. Near-receptors are, of course, also stimulated when, in the delivery of food reinforcers, the teacher places food directly into the child's mouth. In this, the approach bears a resemblance to those of DesLauriers and Carlson (1969), of Zaslow and Breger (1969), and of Schopler (1962); and one wonders whether this common element represents the "effective ingredient" in all these forms of treatment despite their different theoretical bases.

Another way in which stimulation of near-receptors enters into the work of Lovaas can be found in his (controversial) use of painful electric shock. As reported in 1965, Lovaas, Schaeffer, and Simmons were able to modify the behavior of 2 five-year-old identical twins with pronounced autistic features (who had failed to respond to other forms of treatment) by the use of brief, intense electric stimulation. When introduced contingent on the child's self-stimulatory, repetitive, and tantrum behavior, shock came to eliminate this behavior but, in addition, when termination of shock was made contingent on the display of affectionate and approach behaviors, the children learned these adaptive responses toward adults. With children whose atavistic, self-injurious behavior precludes the production of adaptive social responses and with whom other forms of treatment are ineffective, the use of pain as a training device may well be justifiable. DesLauriers and Carlson (1969), who vigorously object to this approach, raise the question whether the affectionate behavior displayed by the twins in the Lovaas study was "true" affection. This, of course, touches on the basic epistemological issue of how one can tell whether a child who smilingly runs toward an adult to hug and kiss him is displaying "real affection." Since an affective state can only be inferred from observed behavior, this issue is ultimately a philosophical one that defies a scientific answer.

Autistic aloneness can be construed as a failure on the part of the child to attend to stimuli emanating from his environment, and an investigator in the behavioral tradition will seek to reduce that deficit. Lovaas, Freitag, Kinder et al. (1966) worked with 2 four-year-old identical twins, schizophrenics "with marked autistic features." While it is not clear whether these were cases of early infantile autism within the narrow definition, the fact that they were identical twins strongly suggests that this was the case since monozygosity is more typical of autism than of schizophrenia (Rimland, 1964). Lovaas and his colleagues, attempting to establish social reinforcement with these children, found that a social stimulus (the word "good") did not acquire reinforcing characteristics along lines of the classical conditioning paradigm. In spite of several hundred trials during which the word was paired with the delivery of food, there was no change in the child's behavior. "Good" had failed to acquire secondary reinforcement properties. The child continued to seem oblivious to the social stimulus; he apparently failed to attend to it. At that time (1966) the authors suggested that failure to attend to social stimuli may be a basic problem of autistic children although Lovaas et al. (1971) have since proposed that *stimulus overselectivity* may be a better explanation of the autistic child's difficulty in classical conditioning.

Having found the classical conditioning paradigm to be ineffective in establishing social reinforcers, Lovaas et al. (1966) turned to the operant model to establish a discriminative social stimulus for the primary reinforcer. That is, the child learned that the presence of the social stimulus (the word "good") signaled the availability of food. Discriminative stimulus training thus forced the child to attend to the social stimulus, not unlike the forcing of attention involved in the intrusive insistence practiced by DesLauriers and Carlson. Given suitable conditions, the autistic child's attention can be established but these conditions must apparently take his high stimulus threshold into consideration. Once Lovaas had established the discrimination (presence of social stimulus = availability of food), he was able to use the social stimulus as an acquired reinforcer to maintain a simple motor response. With intermittent delivery of food, these investigators were able to show that the social stimulus retained its acquired reinforcement property over extended sessions as long as it continued to be discriminative for food.

This study not only supports the assumption that a basic problem of some autistic children centers on their deficient sensitivity to environmental stimuli but it also strengthens the rationale underlying the successful attempts at treating autistic children with operant techniques (e.g., Wetzel, Baker, Roney, & Martin, 1966; Wolf, Risley, Johnston, Harris, & Allen, 1967). These will find more detailed discussion in Chapter 13. Operant approaches view the autistic child as one who has failed to learn socially adaptive response patterns and therapists working in this frame of reference set up systematic contingencies of behavior control designed to build small response units through the immediate use of powerful reinforcers. The intensity of such a regimen appears to be one way of breaking through the autistic child's "stimulus barrier" and "capturing" his attention.

RECAPITULATION

We have seen that the etiologic speculations which have been advanced to explain early infantile autism include propositions dealing with the child's reinforcement history, his cognitive processes, his sensory and affective responsiveness, his ability to establish attachment, his arousal mechanism, and his capacity to select among simultaneous stimuli. Available research does not permit one to decide which of these formulations has the most merit.

When serious investigators examine the same phenomenon but arrive at different conclusions, it is probable that none are entirely wrong and none completely right. As with the blind men examining the elephant, it is likely that the different descriptions derive from the fact that diverse investigators are looking at different aspects of the phenomenon partly, at least, because their theoretical dispositions result in a certain amount of selective perception.

The observed behavioral deficits which form the cluster called *early infantile autism* may very well have a variety or a combination of causes. It seems likely that among these are impairments of such functions as processing sensations and storing memory, hypersensitivity to certain stimulations and hyposensitivity to others, and difficulty in dealing with simultaneous stimuli. In addition, it follows from the principles involved in all other behavioral development that the actions of a child thus impaired interact with the reactions of other people, particularly his parents, to form a highly complex behavior pattern. Given a mother who reacts to an impaired child in a particularly overstimulating, understimulating, or inconsistent manner, the child may develop the characteristics of infantile autism; given a different mother with a different reaction pattern, it is conceivable that the child may develop some other difficulty—maybe the type of learning dysfunction discussed in the next chapter.

5

LEARNING
DIFFICULTIES

As pointed out in Chapter 1, the definition of deviancy in behavior depends on the role expectations a society holds for its members. The role expectation for a child of school age is that he be an adequately performing student. The adequacy of performance is, in turn, defined and evaluated by the school which the child attends in terms of the requirements of that school and the expectations of the community which it serves. In a highly technological, knowledge-oriented society which views education as the key to social mobility and success, inadequate performance in the role of student comes to be viewed as a serious problem by school and family alike. This concern about educational failure has made learning difficulties the one most frequently cited problem of children brought to the attention of professionals concerned with psychological disorders of children (Gilbert, 1957). For reasons to be discussed below it is very difficult to obtain accurate data on the prevalence of school children whose academic performance is below expectations, but informed estimates have placed their number as high as 20 percent of the school-age population (McCarthy & McCarthy, 1969).

THE MEASUREMENT PROBLEM

Learning is a hypothetical construct that refers to a function which can only be inferred from observed changes in performance when they follow certain antecedent events called *training, teaching,* or *experience*. In order to demonstrate this function, one must (among other controls) measure a child's performance before and after an event that one presumes capable of changing (enhancing) his performance. It stands to reason that change should be expected only if the intervening event has relevance for this particular child in his current condition in terms of his developmental level, capacity, and learning history. A gross example may serve to illustrate this point. If, unknown to his teacher, a child were to be totally deaf and the teacher presented him with a verbal statement designed to teach him something, the child would fail to learn. It would make no sense to say that the child has a learning difficulty; it might be more appropriate to say that the difficulty is the teacher's. If, and only if, an appropriate teaching method was used and the child failed to learn, is it then appropriate to say the child has a learning difficulty. Because of this need to assure that the material to be taught and the method by which it is taught are appropriate to the child's condition, the study of learning difficulties encounters problems of major proportions. One can never be certain that a particular teaching method is appropriate as long as a child fails to learn; and the onus is on those who try to teach to exhaust all possible methods before opting for the easy vindication of blaming their teaching failure on the child's learning difficulty (Ross, 1967c).

But the problem of appropriate instruction is not the only complication in this field. Another is the issue of measurement. A learning difficulty represents a discrepancy between a child's estimated academic potential and his actual level of academic performance. This calls not only for a measure of actual performance but also for an index that will permit a valid estimate of potential performance. To determine learning potential one would need a measure of a child's inherent endowment; *there is no such measure*.

The usual mode of estimating a child's learning potential is to analyze his performance on a standard intelligence test. If his score is near the average or above-average range, it is assumed that his potential is at that level; but, as Haring and Bateman (1969) have pointed out, children who fail to score near average on intelligence tests have, upon further examination, been shown to be capable of performance at a higher level. What an intelligence test measures is essentially how much of what the child has learned he is able to display at the time of testing. These tests are, in other words, no more than measures of attainment or achievement and if a child has difficulties in learning, for whatever reasons, this deficit will be reflected in his intelligence test score. A somewhat more sophisticated approach to ascertaining potential than that involved in looking at the overall intelligence test score is the analysis of the relationship of different subtest scores as on such instruments as the Wechsler Intelligence Scale for Children (Wechsler, 1949); but even here the psychologist is only guessing when he assumes the highest subtest scores to reflect the child's "true" potential, particularly in view of the low validity of profile interpretation (Ross, 1959).

There is, as was pointed out, no measure of learning potential, and the intelligence test is a poor substitute. The actual level of performance, with which the presumed "potential" is to be compared in establishing a learning disability, is usually measured by achievement tests so that a statement about learning difficulties is ultimately based on a comparison of scores on two kinds of achievement tests. Since performance on both kinds of tests can be interfered with by the same factors, it is possible that a child shows no discrepancy between his achievement test scores and his intelligence test scores simply because both scores are equally depressed. On the other hand, when a discrepancy does appear, it need not necessarily mean that the child has a learning difficulty; for his difficulty may lie in test performance or in error of measurement or in the previously suggested teaching failure. The dilemma is not solved when the measure of school achievement is based not on test scores but on actual classroom performance, for this only substitutes the unreliability of teachers' grading and often arbitrary promotion policies for the unreliability of formal achievement tests.

Bateman and Schiefelbusch (1969) cogently observe that it is often important to ascertain the general achievement level of a par-

ticular classroom before one can understand why a child's performance is perceived as less than adequate by teacher or parent. If a
child of average intelligence is placed in a class where the mean
ability level is extremely high, he may appear to be performing quite
poorly. On the other hand, it is possible that a severe learning
difficulty remains undetected when a child of very high ability is
placed in a low or low-average classroom or school. These writers
also point out that the significance of a discrepancy between ability
and performance may depend on whether "there is, in fact, something that can be done about the child's achievement problem. If
there is, then the discrepancy is significant and the child has a
learning disability. If there is not, perhaps he should not be so
labeled" (p. 8).

THE TERMINOLOGY

Despite the high incidence of children who are attending school but
not learning, the problem is poorly understood and conceptually unclear. In an attempt to clarify the issues, the National Institute of
Neurological Diseases and Blindness sponsored a 3-phase project
(Clements, 1966, 1969; Chalfant & Scheffelin, 1969) that was to
deal with terminology, services, and research in the area of learning
difficulties. It is a reflection of the ambiguity of the topic that the
three task forces failed to agree on a common terminology. The
group specifically charged with a review of nomenclature recommended the term "minimal brain dysfunction syndrome" and defined
the children under consideration as those "near average, average, or
above average in general intelligence, with certain learning or behavioral disabilities, ranging from mild to severe, which are associated
with deviations of function of the central nervous system" (Clements,
1966, p. 9). The group charged with a discussion of educational
services found this medically oriented definition unacceptable and
preferred instead to speak of "children with learning disabilities" for
whom they offered a definition which stressed that such children
"may or may not show demonstrable deviation in central nervous
system functioning" (Clements, 1969, p. 2). The authors of the
third report, charged with reviewing available research, accepted

neither of these definitions but chose to speak of "central processing dysfunctions in children," pointing out that differences in terminology and definition are to be expected in an area that is of interest to different disciplines, such as education, neurology, pediatrics, and psychology. It may thus be necessary to formulate several definitions, each with relevance for a particular user. "Since the educator must deal with behavior, it may be helpful for the educator to use terms which are descriptive of these behavioral deviations" (Chalfant & Scheffelin, 1969, p. 2).

Like all other labels of psychological disorders, the term *learning difficulties* is no more than a description of what has been observed; it is not an explanation. It is tautological to say that a child has a low score on an achievement test or that he failed to be promoted because he has a learning difficulty. Children may find it difficult to learn for a great variety of reasons. Some may have a limited capacity for academic learning; others may have a sensory impairment. Some may have been deprived of adequate stimulation or early education; others may be emitting responses that are incompatible with learning. Finally, there are those who function in such a manner that the standard teaching methods fail to lead to appropriate learning. It does not further understanding to refer to all of these problems by one label. A somewhat finer discrimination among various forms of learning difficulties can clarify the issues. For this reason we shall focus here the discussion on *learning dysfunctions* (Ross, 1967a) and differentiate these from *learning disorders* and *learning disabilities*.

Learning Disorders

The term *learning disorders* should be reserved to identify those children whose basic capacity to learn is not impaired but whose learning is disrupted or prevented by acquired, incompatible responses. These incompatible responses may be emitted to the stimuli representing specific learning tasks, say reading, or to most stimulus aspects having to do with learning, including school itself. For example, if sitting still and looking at a printed page has acquired aversive properties, the child may learn that he can avoid this condition by moving about and looking away. In instances where reading lessons have been paired with punishment, the printed page may have become a stimulus eliciting anxiety responses, and avoiding the stimulus will then be reinforced by anxiety reduction. For some children, avoidance responses may have generalized to all situations involving learning so that not only one area, such as reading, but the learning of any subject matter is disrupted. Finally, school itself may have become aversive, and the child may refuse to attend school, that is, display the behavior labeled *school phobia*. It will be noted that in each of these instances, the difficulty involves excess behavior, excess anxiety, and excess avoidance responses. For this reason, in the later section dealing with excess behavior, there will be a discussion on school phobia. Children with a learning disorder, as construed here, will display a discrepancy between academic performance and estimated academic potential; and in this fashion they appear the same as children with learning dysfunctions, although the latter, as we shall see, have an entirely different problem involving deficient, rather than excess behavior.

Learning Disabilities

The child with a learning disability will also present a performance-expectation discrepancy, but his problem is of yet another kind. He, too, possesses the functions needed to benefit from academic instruction as ordinarily provided, such as attention, perception, and coordination; but his ability to use these functions is impaired because of psychological disorders that are unrelated to school or learning yet secondarily interfere with or prevent school-appropriate behavior. The observed difficulties in learning and performance are, in these cases, secondary to some other problem, but since a mistaken focus on school performance can lead to confusing such learning disabilities with learning dysfunctions or learning disorders, they merit brief attention. This group includes children with such long-standing and pervasive psychological disorders as infantile autism or childhood schizophrenia which are discussed elsewhere. Suffice it here to point out that the learning ability of these children is almost always severely impaired and the impairment of long standing. In the course of treatment, these children must learn not only the usual academic subject matter but also, and more importantly, such basic self-help and social skills as feeding, dressing, language, and interpersonal behavior. In addition to this group, whose problem might be termed chronic, there is a group of children who, after a period of sustained growth and achievement, begin to fail to perform adequately in school because a temporary, *acute* reaction to stress interferes with their ability to acquire or reproduce academic subject matter. The psychological consequences of the loss of a parent, of having been involved in a frightening accident, or of other sudden, unexpected, and unsettling experiences may temporarily interfere with a child's school performance. Fears associated with leaving the home or the mother, sometimes called *separation anxiety* and often confused with *school phobia*, may be another source of learning disability. In each of these instances, the child is not emitting avoidance responses to school or to learning per se, but he is unable to learn because other reactions militate against learning.

Another group of children should be included under the heading of learning disabilities. These are children who avoid learning or refuse to attend school because these behaviors are reinforced by the attention and concern this elicits from their parents. Where concentrated parental attention can be attained only when the parents are irritated or upset by the child's behavior, this attention is apparently capable of sustaining such self-defeating behavior as not learning or refusing to demonstrate what one has learned by doing well on school tests.

In all of the cases mentioned under the rubric of learning disabilities, the learning difficulty is secondary to other problems, and treatment must address itself to these before the difficulty can be resolved. If effective intervention takes place soon after the onset of the problem which disrupts learning, so that adequate functioning can quickly be restored, the child should be able to continue his academic endeavors without requiring special educational efforts. However, where weeks or months or years have gone by without grade-appropriate learning so that the child has fallen further and further behind his classmates, he will need intensive remedial tutoring, for otherwise fear of failure, censure, or inadequacy may lead to school refusal, thus complicating the picture.

LEARNING DYSFUNCTIONS

When a child does not manifest general mental subnormality, does not show an impairment of visual or auditory functions, is not prevented from attending to his educational tasks by unrelated psychological disorders, and is provided with cultural and educational advantages that are average for his social environment but is nonetheless severely impaired in his learning efficiency, we shall consider him to fall into the category of *learning dysfunctions*. It will be immediately apparent that this is a categorization by exclusion; if the learning difficulty cannot be attributed to any other reason, it is considered a learning dysfunction. It is a reflection of the primitive state of knowledge in this field that every definition in current use focuses on what the condition is *not*, thus begging the question what it *is*.

Children with learning dysfunctions show, upon closer examination, a great variety of difficulties with attention, perception, concept formation, motor control, coordination, and communication. They have been described as hyperactive, distractible, perseverative, impulsive, disoriented, and clumsy. At the level of school performance their impairment may emerge in reading, spelling, arithmetic, or the understanding and production of verbal language. It should be stressed that no child will exhibit all of these difficulties and that no two children will manifest exactly the same pattern.

A great many different labels are currently in use, again reflecting confusion and lack of knowledge about the problem. The children in question are variously said to have learning disabilities, specific learning disabilities, educational handicaps, perceptual handicaps, brain injury, minimal brain damage, or minimal brain dysfunction. It will be noted that the first three terms are essentially descriptive, carrying no explanatory connotations, while the last three imply that the cause for the learning difficulties of these children is to be found in their brain. Attempts to substantiate this neurological hypothesis have so far been unsuccessful (Owen et al., 1971). For some of the children in question a central nervous system dysfunction can indeed be demonstrated, but for most children in this group such terms as minimal brain dysfunction add nothing to the understanding of the problem and largely serve to give the misleading impression that there is a medically identifiable syndrome—and a known (and irreversible) cause of the difficulty.

The assumption of neurological impairment in children who manifest learning dysfunctions is, at least in part, based on the unsound syllogism: Children with learning dysfunctions often display hyperactivity and distractibility; children with demonstrable brain damage often display hyperactivity and distractibility; therefore, children with learning dysfunctions have brain damage, even if it is not otherwise demonstrable. That this reasoning is fallacious was underscored in a careful study by Kasper et al. (1971) who showed that while brain-damaged children are more active and distractible than normal controls in a structured test situation, brain damage does not lead to hyperactivity and distractibility under any and all stimulus conditions "but rather to certain forms of hyperactivity in certain children, certain forms of distractibility in others, and so on" (ibid., p. 337).

At the present time, the reason why some children develop learning dysfunctions remains unknown. Nor is it clear whether some of the behaviors these children exhibit are primary or secondary to other problems. It might be that lack of attention, distractibility, and hyperactivity represent the random response pattern of an aroused organism that has not hit upon the operant that leads to termination of noxious stimulation. In the case of a child this stimulation might be the environmental pressures to acquire expected responses, and the reason for his not emitting the appropriate response might be an inability to perceive the relevant discriminative stimuli or an incapacity to emit the responses in the manner demanded by the environment. On the other hand, lack of attention, distractibility, and hyperactivity might themselves be the reasons why the child is unable to attend to the discriminative stimuli, and so no learning can occur. The latter possibility obviously raises the further question why the child is distractible and hyperactive. When hyperactivity is reduced by either psychological (Patterson, 1965) or pharmacological (Conners, Eisenberg, & Barcai, 1967) means, improvements in the child's ability to learn can be demonstrated, but the effectiveness of a treatment cannot be used to support any particular etiological hypothesis.

While the causal question must be pursued so that learning dysfunctions may ultimately be anticipated and prevented, those charged with helping and teaching children who have a problem in this area can, and must, proceed along pragmatic lines. Help for such children calls neither for inferential speculation nor for profound labels but for imaginative modifications in the educational approach, possibly combined with a sophisticated and controlled administration of certain medications. Perceptual training—in one or more of the sense modalities—the use of perceptual channels other than the visual or auditory, the breaking down of learning tasks into more readily mastered smaller units, and systematic reinforcement programs have, alone or in combination, proved to be successful in helping children overcome or compensate for their learning dysfunction (McLeod, 1967).

Behavioral Assessment

In a behavioral approach, a child's problem in learning is taken as the problem that must be solved. No attempt is made to find "underlying causes" or to speculate about the etiology of the difficulty. Lovitt (1967) outlined four steps essential for such an approach to the assessment of children with learning difficulties. First, the child must be observed over a period of time so that a stable baseline of his school performance can be obtained. If he has problems in reading, this behavior is measured, using such indexes as rate, accuracy, retention, and comprehension. The second step is an assessment of the components of the behavior which has been identified as presenting difficulty. This includes ascertaining relevant stimulus events, as, for example, the child's preference for letter size in the case of reading difficulty; determining the child's responses to the stimuli; finding the contingency system or reinforcement schedule under which the child is operating; and noting the events that follow the child's behavior. If the problem is described as a failure to follow verbal instructions, one should assess such component behaviors as auditory discrimination, immediate auditory memory, attention to auditory stimuli, integration of auditory symbols and visual stimuli, temporal sequencing, and comprehension of structure and function of various linguistic patterns (Bateman & Schiefelbusch, 1969). The third step, following this analysis of the problem behavior, is to involve the referring agent, usually the teacher, to ascertain his or her ability to modify the conditions under which the child is working and to engage this agent's cooperation in the helping procedures to be instituted. The fourth, and last, step in the assessment is to generalize the findings from the assessment situation to the day-to-day classroom conditions since, knowing how the child reads, his reading behavior can now be modified. With the kind of specific suggestions possible on the basis of such a behavioral analysis, the teacher is able to institute concrete changes that are designed to help the child overcome his problem.

The assessment of learning dysfunctions is often complicated by a child's secondary psychological reactions to the pressures represented by puzzled, frustrated, and anxious parents or teachers who cannot understand the discrepancy between the child's intelligence level and scholastic achievement. The child's reactions may take various forms, such as avoidance, escape, or attack responses and when these are viewed as the cause rather than the effect of the learning problem, treatment efforts may be misdirected and, hence, ineffective. A child may not be able to learn and, consequently, become anxious. This anxiety may further reduce his capacity to learn or to perform what he has learned, thus setting up a vicious cycle and complicating the assessment process.

Help for children who manifest secondary psychological reactions to learning dysfunctions calls not only for the introduction of special educational techniques but also for attention to the confounding secondary reaction. Both efforts must be coordinated and carefully paced if they are to be effective. For example, a child who has developed a fear of failure as a result of repeated failure experiences in his academic endeavors is unlikely to benefit from special education until he can face learning tasks without their eliciting avoidance responses. He will also need to acquire some degree of confidence in his own abilities, and he is unlikely to gain such confidence until he has had some success experiences. Learning tasks must therefore be so arranged that the child can be sure of experiencing repeated success. Since this is the principle that underlies programmed learning using so-called teaching machines, such programs, used in conjunction with reinforcement principles, have been successfully applied in complex cases of learning difficulties (e.g., Staats & Butterfield, 1965).

Sensory—Motor Integration

Among the steps in assessment outlined by Lovitt (1967) is the need to ascertain relevant stimulus events and the child's responses to these stimuli. Almost all of the stimulus events presented to a child by the school situation are in the visual or auditory realm, and the responses to be emitted by the child are largely in the motor realm, as in the production of spoken or written verbal or quantitative language. Most learning dysfunctions, particularly those identified in the primary grades, thus emerge along the sensory input-motor output process, an observation reflected in the term *sensory-motor dysfunction* which has had wide currency in the literature on learning difficulties. The usual implication (Kephart, 1960) is that the source of the difficulty is in the child's inability to perform the function necessary to relate sensory stimuli to motor responses. As with other inferences about central processes it has been difficult to study sensory-motor integration objectively.Their review of research in this area led Chalfant and Scheffelin (1969) to the conclusion that attempts to demonstrate the correlation between reading failure and such variables as laterality, visual perception, or integration have had conflicting results.

Occasionally a study demonstrates a relationship between reading difficulty and some other functions such as finger localization (Croxen & Lytton, 1971), but the meaning of such findings, either in causal or remedial terms, remains unclear. Beery (1967), for example, explored the ability of average and retarded readers to match auditory and visual stimuli. In this study fifteen children, whose reading achievement was at least 2 years below the age-appropriate grade level, were matched for intelligence test scores, age, and sex with a control group of normal readers. All the children were within the normal range of tested intelligence. The experimental tasks required that they match visually presented patterns of dots with an analogous pattern of discrete, recorded tones coming from a speaker and vice versa. In one test, the auditory stimuli were presented first, followed by the visual patterns; in a second test the presentation was reversed. The test pattern was presented, and after it had been withdrawn, the child had to recognize the correct representation from among three choices in the case of the auditory-visual sequence, two in the visual-auditory sequence. The task thus involved not only matching but also immediate recall and, of course, attention. The results showed that on both series the normal controls performed significantly better than the retarded readers, thus confirming earlier findings by Birch and Belmont (1964). Further research is needed to determine whether retarded readers have difficulty on these matching tasks because they do not attend to the stimuli, fail to recall the stimulus pattern, find visual stimuli aversive, are unmotivated to give correct responses, or cannot, indeed, relate stimuli from two different sense modalities. From a predictive and remedial standpoint it would be important to know whether the difficulty on matching tasks of this nature can be detected in pre-school children before the reading difficulty becomes identified and whether, where remedial reading is successfully applied, the auditory-visual matching performance improves.

A study conducted at the University of Arkansas Medical Center (Dykman et al., 1970) indicates that children with learning difficulties take longer to process information than their unimpaired peers. These investigators compared the reaction times of eighty-two boys described as "working below capacity in one or more basic subjects" with those of thirty-four controls who were "academically adequate." The nonspecific, largely judgmental basis of subject selection is one of the weaknesses of this study. Nonetheless, it is worth noting the finding that on a simple task requiring the child to press a key upon presentation of a stimulus light, those with school-learning problems had mean response latencies of 558 milliseconds, while the mean for the control group was 466 milliseconds. If this difference is statistically significant (the authors fail to report a relevant data analysis) and if the results can be replicated in a more rigorously controlled experiment, the suggestion that teachers of children with learning difficulties should speak more slowly and repeat their messages so as to accommodate to the slower "thinking time" of their students might be worthy of consideration.

In many of the studies and observations of children with learning dysfunctions their problem with attention is a recurrent theme. In recent years attention has received increasing consideration in the research and theoretical formulations of a great many psychologists (Mostofsky, 1970). Many view attention as related to or synonymous with arousal; defective attention may thus be similar to defective arousal. If we recall that defective arousal was implicated in early infantile autism by several of the investigators discussed in Chapter 4, it may now be apparent why we concluded that chapter with a speculation about a relationship between early infantile autism and learning dysfunctions.

Remedial Work

Remedial work with children whose learning dysfunction is most pronounced in reading has often been guided by one or the other etiologic speculation. Thus, those who subscribe to the notion of a developmental failure in establishing perceptual-motor integration have attempted to recapitulate early phases of motor development or to give so-called perceptual-motor training. Some highly publicized versions of these approaches have elicited a good deal of public interest, but there is "little empirical evidence that would support the contention that basic perceptual-motor training leads to improvement in perceptual-motor abilities or to better academic performance" (Chalfant & Scheffelin, 1969, p. 28).

When reading is viewed as operant behavior and analyzed in terms of its component tasks, highly successful remedial approaches can be demonstrated (Goldiamond & Dyrud, 1966). Using minimally trained adult volunteers and high school seniors as therapy technicians, Staats, Minke, Goodwin, and Landeen (1967) accelerated the reading rate of eighteen junior high school students who had been retarded readers. The desired responses were reinforced with small amounts of money, the amount per reading response being reduced as the reading rate accelerated and the material became more difficult.

The matter of using extrinsic reinforcers to improve reading behavior received systematic investigation in a study conducted by Sibley (1966). One of the major purposes of this research was to evaluate the possibility of employing conditioned reinforcers to increase the tendency of a child to make a reading response. Seven second-grade children of normal intelligence, who had been evaluated as poor readers, were the subjects. Their total reading responses was the dependent variable, while the type of reinforcer (tokens or points) was the primary independent variable. The effectiveness of points was assessed when they were presented alone; they were then paired with the tokens that could be traded for selected backup reinforcers, and finally, the points were again presented alone to determine any change in reinforcing effectiveness. The schedule on which the tokens were delivered was varied, ranging from continuous reinforcement to FR30. The results of the study indicated that the reinforcement conditions had a significant effect on total responding. The points were originally not reinforcing, but became "strikingly powerful reinforcers" (p. 4135) after pairing with tokens. Analysis of individual performance curves showed that the less successful, less persevering, and less productive subjects performed best under lower ratios, such as FR2, while the generally more able subjects performed better at high ratios. The study thus not only demonstrates that points, an easily applicable conditioned reinforcer, can be made effective when they are first paired with a more concrete generalized reinforcer; it also underscores that reinforcement schedules must be individualized if they are to be maximally effective in helping poor readers learn to read.

An important aspect of learning dysfunctions and other learning difficulties is that they represent a cumulatively worsening process owing to the pyramidal nature of education. A child who has been unable to learn the basic tool subjects in the primary grades experiences an ever increasing disability, since later teaching is always based on competencies presumed to have been established earlier. Concomitantly, continued exposure to the situations in which the child is expected to learn but encounters failure will make these situations ever more aversive and hence ever more likely to elicit escape or avoidance behavior. In 1967 Coleman and Sandhu published a report describing 364 children with learning difficulties who had been referred to a clinic specializing in these problems. They pointed out that 41 percent of these children were 2 or more years behind in their school work by the time they were brought to the clinic. It is also of interest that in this group boys outnumbered girls 6 to 1. Similar ratios are reported from other sources, suggesting either that boys tend to encounter greater difficulty under the prevailing educational system or that parents and teachers are more readily concerned when a boy rather than a girl exhibits problems in learning. In view of the possible relationship between learning difficulties and other behavior problems of boys to which Miller, Hampe, Barrett, and Noble (1971) have called our attention (see Chapter 2), the importance of early detection and immediate remediation of learning dysfunctions cannot be given enough stress.

RECAPITULATION

Despite their prevalence and the degree of concern they occasion, learning difficulties are a form of psychological disorder that is poorly understood. Problems in measurement and confusion in definition have contributed to this state of affairs. A finer discrimination among various forms of learning difficulties might clarify the issues. For this reason learning disorders, learning disabilities, and learning dysfunctions were given separate discussions. Children with learning dysfunctions are often described as having poor motor control and low attention spans and as being hyperactive and impulsive. These characteristics have led some to speculate that these children might have a central nervous system dysfunction, but such a neurological hypothesis has never been proven. For those charged with helping these children, etiologic speculations are largely irrelevant. They must ask the question what the child needs to learn and then proceed to teach him by carefully individualized methods. Such a pragmatic approach has been shown to be successful in many cases. As we shall see in the next chapter, such an approach also works with children who "everyone has always known" could not possibly learn anything—the profoundly retarded.

6

MENTAL SUBNORMALITY

The psychological disorder to be discussed in this chapter has had various labels, including *mental retardation, mental deficiency, amentia,* and *feeblemindedness.* Each of these labels has reference to inadequate mental processes whose presence can only be inferred by observing a child's inadequate performance. We examined the logical and methodological problems that are encountered when one resorts to such inferences in the previous chapter. Largely because of these problems, the realm of mental subnormality, no less than that of learning difficulties, is fraught with controversy. When a child's observed performance falls short of some arbitrary standard, this inadequacy may have a host of reasons—only one of which might be a permanent defect in his mental processes.

The arbitrary standard with which a child's performance is compared is inevitably a reflection of the expectations his society holds about what is appropriate performance for a child at his chronological age. In other words, if, in comparison with other children his age, his performance is deemed deficient and he approaches the tasks in a manner considered appropriate for children at a younger developmental level, he is called *retarded.* On tests that have been developed in order to make the comparison between a child's performance and that of his peers more uniform—that is, tests of intelligence—this type of child achieves a significantly lower score than the norm for his age, hence the term *mental subnormality.*

The observations based on test performance are usually expressed in a numerical code, the intelligence quotient (IQ). This tends to obscure two important points which must be kept in mind in any discussion of mental subnormality. The first point is that whatever deficiency may find expression in the test score, it is no more than a deficiency in observable behavior, including test behavior. Any reference to mental processes represents an inference, an allusion to a construct for which we have, at the present time, no independent, nonbehavioral criterion. The observed deficiency is undoubtedly present in the behavior of many children, whether the deficiency is *mental* remains a speculation. Bijou (1966) once suggested that a term more in keeping with a natural-science approach than mental retardation would be *developmental retardation.* This is purely descriptive and makes no assumptions about unobservable mental processes. Unfortunately, Bijou's suggestion has not been taken up by other writers in this field, and since the traditional terminology has greater currency, it will be used in these pages but with the understanding that the word *mental* is merely a conventional code that stands for the various observable behaviors traditionally considered to be manifestations of mental processes.

The second point to be underscored is that mental subnormality is a performance deficit and not a disease entity. The judgment of subnormality or retardation is inevitably a relative, social judgment, made in the context of the child's social environment and the demands that environment places upon him. Tests of intelligence, though standardized and objective in the sense that they can be scored according to a uniform norm, are no more than a codification of the kinds of behaviors a given society considers important at its time in history.

DEFINITION

Both of the above points find consideration in the definition of mental retardation advanced by the American Association on Mental

Deficiency (AAMD) (Heber, 1959; revised 1961) which states that "mental retardation refers to subaverage general intellectual functioning which originates during the developmental period and is associated with impairment in adaptive behavior" (Heber, 1961, p. 3). In elaboration of this definition, the AAMD publication states that "general intellectual functioning" is assessed by the use of tests and that "impairment in adaptive behavior" may be reflected in maturation, learning, and/or social adjustment. Since maturation, learning, and social adjustment are of different importance at different age levels, an individual may satisfy the definition of mental retardation at one time in his life but not at another. As a result of changes in social standards or conditions, or as a result of changes in his own efficiency of functioning, an individual's status may change since his level of functioning must always be "determined in relation to the behavioral standards and norms" for his age group (ibid. 1961, p.4).

It is important to recognize that this view of mental retardation avoids the notion of a permanent, immutable state and that it makes no assumption about the cause of this behavioral deficit. When a child fails to give correct answers to the questions on an intelligence test, he may do so for one of several reasons or because of a combination of these reasons. The most obvious of these reasons is that he has never been taught the responses expected of him. On the Wechsler Intelligence Scale for Children (WISC) (Wechsler, 1949), for example, there appear such questions as "Where does the sun set?" and "At 7 cents each, what will 3 cigars cost?" The average ten-year-old is expected to answer these questions correctly. A child who has never attended school or whose school is so inadequate that he has never had an opportunity to learn the answers to these and similar questions will in all likelihood be unable to give the correct response; and his test score, when converted into IQ points, may well fall into the subaverage range, defined as one standard deviation below the population mean for his age group. Children whose subnormal functioning is the result of poor schooling and similar environmental factors, the *culturally disadvantaged*, are severely handicapped in a highly competitive, technological urban society. It is obvious that corrective measures for this condition must take the form of massive compensatory education and drastic improvement in educational opportunities. It is also obvious that the subnormal functioning of such children need not be a permanent condition and that their impairment in adaptive behavior is relative to certain social demands (school performance) and not to others (finding one's way on city streets).

Another reason why a child's intelligence-test performance may fall in the subnormal range may be that while he was exposed to opportunities for acquiring the expected skills around the same time as other children his age, he failed to learn them. Some children may learn these skills from months to years later than their age group; others may never master them. Those who acquire appropriate skills more slowly than their peers, whose development is retarded, might appropriately be called *mentally retarded* while those who are incapable of acquiring these skills altogether might be categorized as *mentally defective.* This distinction was advanced by Masland, Sarason, and Gladwin (1958), but like all labels, these terms are inadequate and beg a great many questions. What, for example, happens to the label when a child whose mental development had been retarded slows down more and then fails to make further progress? Does he cease being mentally retarded and become mentally defective?

The term "defective" implies that there is some defect in the child, that he is of limited potential or capacity, and that—no matter what one might try—he would be unable to acquire additional skills. The term "retardation" merely states an observation: The child is less advanced than his peers. The term "defective," on the other hand, carries implications of a limited potential. Potential, representing a projection into the future, can never be known; it can only be guessed and, given presently available tools, this guess is most hazardous. At best, one can make the statement that at the time and in the manner a given skill was taught, such a child did not learn it. The stress must be on present behavior and not on uncertain estimates of potential and future functioning. With that, the focus is placed not on the child's learning capacity but on the manner in which teaching is attempted.

Whether it be tying a shoelace; acquiring language; learning to read, write, or do arithmetic, the culture and its educational system generally make the assumption that all children can and should master these skills under the same conditions and in the same manner. Elementary school, in particular, operates on the unwarranted assumption that one mode of teaching is optimal for all of the children in a given class. The child who fails to learn reading, writing, spelling, or arithmetic is assumed to have "something wrong with him." The problem is seen as *his* learning problem, not as his school's teaching problem. He is then usually given an intelligence test (which relies heavily on questions involving things one learns in school), and when he attains a low score, this "explains" why he has failed to learn : he is mentally retarded. The fact that this description is not an explanation is ignored, and the possibility that this particular child might have been able to learn if a different mode of teaching had been used is rarely, if ever, considered.

CLASSIFICATION

Since mental subnormality is a matter of degree, intelligence test scores and their standard deviation have been used to establish subclassifications. According to the American Association on Mental Deficiency (Heber, 1959), scores from tests like the Wechsler Intelligence Scale for Children divide the range of mental subnormality as follows :

Level of Retardation	IQ Score Range
Borderline	70-84
Mild	55-69
Moderate	40-54
Severe	25-39
Profound	under 25

Such a classification is, of course, no more than an assignment of verbal labels to ranges of test scores, ranges based on the statistical concept of one standard deviation. That is, scores between one and two standard deviations below the mean are called *borderline*, between two and three standard deviations, *mild*, and so forth. It is important to stress the arbitrary nature of these classifications. It is meaningless to call a child with an IQ score of 54 "moderately retarded" while with a score of 55 he would be called "mildly retarded." This is particularly apparent when one recalls that the standard error of measurement of most intelligence tests is around five points.

The issue is further complicated by the fact that the test scores and labels traditionally used in the area of mental subnormality are not merely statements describing observed facts but statements from which people draw inferences about the child's future behavior, about his "potential." The inferential implications of IQ scores have found expression in the terms *trainable*, applied to children with scores between roughly 25 and 49, and *educable*, describing those with scores above 50 but below 76. The educable are expected to be able to do academic work at least to the third-grade level, occasionally to the sixth-grade level, by the time they are sixteen years old. The trainable, on the other hand, are not expected to master academic skills. The goal of training for the latter is to teach them self-care and to cope with simple routines under supervision. Used in this manner, the test scores carry clear implications of potential.

When a young child's measured intelligence quotient is 45, this not only means that he now functions at the level of moderate retardation, it also suggests to many psychologists and educators that he will be unable to benefit from academic instruction since his "potential" is viewed as below the expectations of elementary school (as presently constituted). A test score reflects present performance; it is not a measure of future potential. Yet once a child's present performance is measured and recorded, the inference about his potential often becomes a self-fulfilling prophecy. Because of his low score he will be excluded from elementary school. What training he receives will be gauged to his presumed capacity, and the end result will be that he does not learn such academic subject matter as reading and arithmetic—just as his test score had "predicted."

Estimates of potential for children in the subnormal range of intelligence are extremely hazardous; unless they are continuously questioned, they are likely to lead to standardized training procedures that are deemed successful when they permit a child to function at the level of his predicted potential. If one takes a low IQ score for what it is—a measure of present performance—and makes no assumptions about limited future potential, one is led to a continuous search for different training and teaching methods for each individual child, expecting that one can help him raise his present level of performance. In settings where preconceptions about limited potential are discarded, as in the program described by Birnbrauer, Wolf, Kidder, and Tague (1965), retarded children can achieve at levels previously thought "impossible." It is a salutary development that terms like trainable and educable as well as some of the more rigid uses of other classifications in the field of mental subnormality are beginning to be discarded.

ETIOLOGY

A great deal has been written about the cause or etiology of *mental subnormality* because it is hoped that knowing how this condition develops will permit its prevention. The trouble with that hope is that mental subnormality is not *a condition*, analogous to a disease; it is a term which describes observable behavior (i.e., behavior measured by an intelligence test). A low score on an intelligence test, in and of itself, says nothing about etiology. An intelligence test score is no more than a statement of how a child's test performance compares to the performance of other children his age. Relative to those other children a child's score may be higher or lower; why it is higher or lower is not revealed by the quantitative statement. If it is significantly lower, the child may be said to be mentally subnormal because his score is below the *normal*, but to say that his score is low *because* he is mentally subnormal would be a fallacious circularity.

In order to discuss the possible meaning that might be attributed to a low intelligence test score, it is well to turn to a brief examination of how these scores are distributed. Measured intelligence is a complex function of the interaction of many genetic and environmental factors. *If* these factors were subject only to random variation, their interaction would generate the well-known bell-shaped curve of normal distribution. But such random variation does not take place. The variation of heredity is constrained by social obstacles to random breeding, and the variation of environment is constrained by the fact that social obstacles prevent random assignment of any individual to any environment. What is more, these social constraints are particularly potent in matters directly related to intelligence. The girl of high intelligence is likely to attend college where the choice of potential mates is biased in favor of intelligent boys, and the child of such a union is likely to be raised in an intellectually stimulating environment. Since the converse is likely to be true in the case of the girl of low intelligence, the actual picture is more that of selective breeding with selective assignment of environment than of random variation of factors.

The *normal* distribution of intelligence along a single, continuous, bisymmetrical curve is a theoretical ideal that probably bears little relationship to reality. It should be noted that it is impossible to ascertain the actual shape of this distribution given only existing tests of intelligence with which to conduct such an investigation. All standardized tests of intelligence are constructed on the assumption of normal distribution of "intelligence." Questions are carefully selected so that only a predetermined percentage of children at each age level will pass the items, and this percentage reflects the test constructor's theoretical assumption about the normal distribution of the construct he is trying to measure. Once test standardization is completed, the scores will generally distribute along the bell-shaped curve simply because that was the goal of the standardization. A test that failed to give a normal distribution of scores would be rejected as invalid; the validity of the underlying assumption is rarely questioned.

Leaving aside the question of the validity of the assumption of a normal distribution of intelligence, whatever the actual shape of the distribution that may be generated by the polygenic model and the nonrandom influences mentioned earlier, there are children whose intellectual development is disrupted by inborn or acquired physical damage or defect. The low intelligence of these children contributes disproportionately to the low end of the distribution of intelligence scores, further distorting its bisymmetry. A number of writers (Dingman & Tarjan, 1960; Penrose, 1963; Zigler, 1967) have pointed out that the low end of the distribution has many more cases than the theoretical normal curve would predict, and some have spoken of a "pathological bulge" in the curve representing the scores of retardates with physical defects whose extremely low scores, largely in the IQ range below 50, occur with disproportionate frequency.

Familial Retardation

Zigler (1967) advocates a two-group approach to mental retardation, stating that the polygenic model of intelligence generates a distribution from IQ 50 to 150. In such a distribution some individuals will be expected to have scores considerably above the mean, while the scores of others should be considerably below the mean. Those at this lower end of the range are viewed as individuals whose low intelligence is an expression of the same factors that contribute to *normal* intelligence. In Zigler's approach these form one group, the *familial retardates*, who represent about 75 percent of all retardates. Their intelligence scores fall roughly between 50 and 70, and they do not have demonstrable physical defects. The other group, whose scores range from 0 to 70—with a mean of approximately 35—do have physical, "organic" defects which severely impair their intellectual functioning. They are "abnormal" in the usual sense of that word in that their scores are not a part of the normal distribution. Zigler's view is illustrated in Figure 6.

According to that view, the familial retardate is *normal* in the statistical sense; his score is an integral part of the dispersion of intelligence test scores that one would predict from the manifestations of the gene pool in a population.

Within such a framework it is possible to refer to the familial retardate as less intelligent than other normal manifestations of the genetic pool, but he is just as integral a part of the normal distribution as are the 3 percent of the population

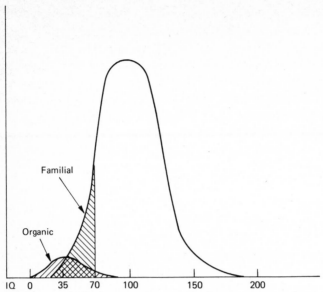

Fig. 6. Distribution of intelligence test scores according to Zigler's two-group approach. (After Zigler, 1967.)

whom we view as superior, or the more numerous group of individuals whom we consider to be average [Zigler, 1967, p. 293].

The familial retardate usually comes from a family where many relatives also score in the subnormal range of intelligence. While genetic factors undoubtedly contribute to this low level of functioning, it would be erroneous to conclude that hereditary factors are solely responsible. Parents of low intelligence not only transmit to their children their limited genetic endowment but they also provide them with an intellectually impoverished environment.

Organic Retardation

While familial retardates come largely from the retarded segment of the population, and tend to score in the mild to borderline range of subnormality, children with physiological defects come from families at all levels of socioeconomic status and measured intelligence. Their defect is presumably caused by an accidental factor and not, as in the case of the familial defectives, by a combination of several adverse conditions. Organic retardation may be due to a single recessive gene, as in the case of gargoylism, amaurotic idiocy, or phenylketonuria. The latter disorder, usually referred to as PKU, has received rather wide publicity although it occurs only about once in 10,000 live births (Robinson & Robinson, 1965). The interest in this condition stems from the fact that it represents one of the few types of severe mental retardation whose genetic-metabolic cause is well enough understood that preventive measures have become possible. Since these children have a metabolism that is incapable of transforming the protein substance phenylalanine, resulting in the release of phenylpyruvic acid into the body, ultimate injury to the brain and the resulting mental retardation can be prevented by placing the child on a diet that is low in phenylalanine.

Even in cases where the etiology is clearly identified and reducible to a single recessive gene, as in PKU, it would be a mistake to assume that the children who are afflicted with that condition form a homogeneous group of retardates. The degree of retardation varies with PKU children; and, as Steisel, Friedman, and Wood (1967) have shown, PKU children are a heterogeneous group in terms of their social interaction so that, behaviorally, *phenylketonuria* is not a unitary disorder.

Another type of mental retardation, *mongolism* or *Down's Syndrome*, has been found to be related to a chromosomal defect. This takes the form of a third chromosome 21, an error in cell division apparently having taken place during formation of the ovum and before conception. For reasons not yet understood, this occurs with greater frequency in older than in younger parents. While it is a disorder involving genetic material, trisomy-21 mongolism is not hereditary, suggesting that environmental changes related to aging may play a significant role. Other severe organic retardation, where the damage is clearly caused by environmental factors, is found in children whose mothers had received radiation treatment while pregnant, in cases of Rh incompatibility, in congenital syphilis, encephalitis, maternal rubella during pregnancy, lead poisoning, and accidental injury to the brain.

BRAIN INJURY

It is a reasonably safe assumption that intellectual processes take place in the brain. Hence the source of impairment of these processes should be located in the brain. This reasoning has led many researchers in the field of mental retardation to speak of brain-injured (organic) and non-brain-injured (familial) retardates and to seek methods for the differentiation between the two groups. Such differentiation is rather easy when a child is profoundly retarded, for here one usually finds such characteristic physical stigmata as those of gargoylism, mongolism, microcephaly, or hydrocephaly. It is in the IQ range from 50 to 70, where organic and familial cases overlap (see Figure 6) that differentiation is difficult if not impossible, given currently available tools.

A large-scale study that attempted to differentiate between brain-injured and so-called garden variety, or non-brain-injured children was conducted by Birch, Belmont, Belmont, and Taft (1967) who examined all educable mentally retarded children aged 8, 9, and 10 living in the city of Aberdeen, Scotland. The WISC was administered, and the test patterns were compared with independent evidence of central nervous system damage. Finding no association, these authors concluded that available psychometric evidence does not support the view that patterns of intellectual functioning are systematically associated with brain damage and that on this basis it is not possible to designate educable mentally subnormal children as "brain-damaged" or "non-brain-damaged." They suggest that either the WISC is insensitive to these etiologic refinements or that the whole range of educable retarded children are children with brain defects. This sweeping conclusion ignores a third possible explanation, namely, that all these children have had similar reinforcement histories so that they displayed similar behavior when given the intelligence test. At any rate, it does not appear very productive to seek etiologic differentiation between retarded children with the test pattern of the Wechsler scale.

It could be argued that a single test of intelligence cannot possibly discriminate between brain-damaged mentally retarded children and non-brain-damaged mentally retarded children. It is thus instructive to examine the results of a research effort that brought a great variety of tests to bear on the question of differential diagnosis. The large-scale, 7-year-long Ability Structure Project directed by Johs Clausen (1966) had among its aims to differentiate the mentally retarded into subgroups which are psychologically and behaviorally more homogeneous than those provided by existing classification systems. The project further sought to relate the factors underlying these subgroupings "to etiology as presumed from medical and family history" (p. 5). In addition, Clausen proposed "to provide the raw material which may make possible the development of new diagnostic tools and to provide new ways of combining results of existing tests to achieve maximum diagnostic power" (loc. cit.).

The project used 388 children from six institutions who were tested on 33 tasks ranging from psychophysical measures, such as 2-point threshold and brightness discrimination, to such intelligence tests as the Porteus Mazes and Thurstone's Test of Primary Mental Abilities. On the basis of their histories and medical records the children were classified into groups of *familials, organics, mixed, mongoloids, unexplained,* and *not classifiable.* All were given a neurological examination and an EEG. The data were then subjected to analysis of variance, correlational analysis, traditional factor analysis, inverse factor analysis, and what the author calls a "syndrome analysis." The published report on the project covers more than 200 pages.

In terms of its aims, the results of this massive effort were singularly disappointing. The relevant conclusions are summarized as follows: "The differentiation of the mentally retarded into subgroups . . . has not been particularly successful. The outline of some broad groups has been presented, but well-defined, specific groups have not been encountered" (p. 172). "The finding of relationship between configuration of abilities and extent of central nervous system damage . . . has been only moderately successful" (p. 173). "With limited success in defining homogeneous subgroups, the attempt to demonstrate relationships between these groups and traditional etiological groups have not been very productive," and "it can hardly be said that new diagnostic tools have been developed. . ." (ibid.).

The results—or lack of results—of this ambitious project would seem to lend support to the contention that attempts to group mental retardates either in terms of ability or in terms of etiology are misdirected and unproductive. No currently available psychological test can differentiate among the traditional etiologic groupings, and new groupings do not emerge from sophisticated statistical analyses. Not even the much-used dichotomy of organic and familial held up in Clausen's study, leading him to conclude that

> It is possible that mild organic impairment is of similar nature to the functional impairment of incomplete development which occurs in the familial retardate. The consequences of this would be that the etiological distinction into familials and organics, at least of the milder cases, has limited significance, as it does not reflect behavioral differences (p. 165f).

An extensive battery of available tests thus fails to permit one to differentiate between retarded children in terms of presence or absence of brain injury. Even if such differentiation were readily accomplished, the knowledge thus gained would hardly aid in making plans for helping an individual child. It may thus be well to turn our attention to other, more pragmatic questions.

THE REINFORCEMENT HISTORY OF THE MENTALLY SUBNORMAL

The mentally subnormal child, by definition, functions at a less than adequate level of adaptation. This fact will color all of his interactions with his environment, and it will therefore influence his general pattern of behavior. This impact of impairment in adaptive behavior on the psychological development of the child would be the same regardless of whether the impairment is due to "organic" or "familial" reasons. If the experiences of these children are similar, no matter what the etiology of their retardation, they would acquire a response repertoire that would make them, as a group, more similar than different by the time they are tested at age eight, as was the case in Clausen's (1966) study.

It is a well-established finding (Zigler, 1966a) that when retarded and normal children are matched on mental age, the retarded perform less well or differently than the normal on many learning and problem-solving tests. Matching for mental age presumably equates intellectual functioning; remaining differences in performance are therefore thought to be due to other than intellectual factors. Those who hold, what Zigler (1960) has called, the "difference orientation" maintain that the familial retardate represents an inherently different type of organism who suffers from a basic defect in either physiological or cognitive structure. This defect is thought to be responsible for the child's impaired performance. The support for this position has been evaluated by Zigler (1966a), who is led to reject this view in favor of a motivational or developmental orientation. When, for purposes of research, one matches a ten-year-old child who functions at the mental age of seven (IQ 70) with a seven-year-old child who also functions at the mental age of seven (IQ 100), one may have matched test performance expressed in a mental-age score; but one has not matched reinforcement history, for, if nothing else, the retardate has lived 3 years longer. Moreover, these 3 years have been filled with failure experiences, as have all the other years of his life.

With this reasoning in mind, it is perhaps significant that the key variables in Clausen's (1966) test battery that differentiated between the retarded and the normal (though not between brain-injured and familial) were pure tone threshold and such simple motor tasks, as lower-arm movement and reaction time. Approaching these findings from the standpoint of a difference theorist, Clausen sees these tests as reflecting the retardates' impairment of such general factors as arousal, vigilance, effort, and response initiation and—without any physiological evidence whatever—attributes this impairment to the ascending reticular activating system in the brainstem. A more parsimonious explanation would seem to be that the retarded children have learned not to trust their judgment or to initiate responses on their own initiative: attributes that are essential for adequate performance on pure tone discrimination, reaction time, and simple motor-task experiments. Zigler (1966a) views such performance deficit as reflecting the retardate's learned "outer-directed response style."

According to Zigler (1966a), this outer-directed style of problem solving is acquired in the often repeated situation where the child is selectively reinforced for careful attentiveness to external cues. When, on the other hand, he bases a response on his own meager cognitive resources, he almost invariably encounters negative consequences. He thus comes to acquire an overreliance on external cues—an outer-directedness, as Zigler would have it. As this outer-directedness generalizes, the child would come to attend in rapid succession to a wide variety of stimuli. His behavior would then be characterized as "distractible," a characteristic that has often been attributed to the retarded child and has, in fact, been viewed by some as an inherent characteristic—basic deficit—of the retarded and as an indication of brain injury.

While this learned behavioral characteristic tends to interfere with the problem-solving ability of retarded children because they attend to misleading and distracting cues (Achenbach & Zigler, 1968), Turnure and Zigler (1964) have shown that retarded children's problem solving can be enhanced when extraneous stimuli are task-relevant or if, as Zeaman and House (1963) have pointed out, these stimuli increase attention by introducing novelty.

Investigators like Zeaman and House (1963), who have carried on extensive studies of various aspects of discrimination learning using retarded subjects, frequently point to deficits in attention-directing ability as a crucial factor in the poor performance of retarded children. When children of different mental ages are compared, those with lower mental age take considerably longer to attend to the relevant task dimensions. Once they attend to these dimensions, however, the children do not differ in their *rate* of learning the discrimination. Attending to the cues an experimenter considers relevant to his task would seem to be another learned form of behavior. An environment that does not provide sufficient opportunities for such learning for a child who learns more slowly than the normal may well provide the basis for developing an attention deficit. Again, it would seem to be unnecessary to postulate inherent, hence irreversible, defects in some inferred "attending mechanism." The presence of such an inherent defect in all retardates is particularly unlikely in view of the fact that investigators who study discrimination learning in institutions for the retarded rarely differentiate among their subjects in terms of familial and organic factors. When these different etiologic groups show a common deficit, it is far more parsimonious to look for the source of this deficit in common conditions of learning than in common structural impairment.

LEARNING BY THE MENTALLY SUBNORMAL

The research evidence mentioned so far supports the contention that the classification of the retarded in terms of presumed etiologies is neither feasible, using present-day psychological tools, nor necessary in terms of educational planning. As Birch et al. (1967) pointed out, the etiologic designation of brain damage does not lead to a clearly defined educational strategy, and so an assessment of the educational capacities and incapacities of a particular child is a more useful basis for a program of training than knowing whether he should be called *brain-damaged* or *familial*.

Not only does it seem irrelevant to know the etiology of a child's maladaptive behavior but it also appears unnecessary to be too concerned with classification into intellectual categories, that is, by IQ test scores. Support for this statement can be found in the rapidly growing literature that shows that the basic principles of learning operate at all levels of intelligence.

From the point of view of the applicability of learning principles, there are no inherent differences between the normal and the retarded, regardless of degree of retardation. Certainly, genetic and physiological conditions set limits on the speed of acquisition and on a child's ultimate response repertoire, but learning can take place and does take place according to the same principles whether the learner be profoundly or mildly retarded. Kingsley (1968), for example, demonstrated that on an associative-learning task a group of educable mentally retarded children performed in a qualitatively similar manner as other ability groups, while Morgan (1969) showed that there is no difference in responsiveness to stimulus complexity at different levels of intelligence. As Ullman and Krasner (1969) have stated, not even the most severe defect rules out responses to the environment and alteration of behavior through training. From this point of view it makes no sense to differentiate between the trainable and the educable—a pseudo-classification which, we must remind ourselves, is simply another arbitrary cutoff on the continuum of intelligence test scores that is no more valid than the discarded idiot, imbecile, moron trichotomy.

A demonstration of the applicability of principles of learning at even the most profound level of retardation can be found in the work of Bailey and Meyerson (1969). These investigators worked with a seven-year-old boy who was blind and at least partially deaf. He had no speech or language, was not toilet trained, and could neither feed himself nor walk. Virtually his entire waking hours were taken up with such stereotyped behaviors as slapping his face; hitting himself on the chin, ears, and side of the head; sucking on his fingers or whole hand; and banging his head, teeth, or a foot against the bars of his crib. Having installed a leather-padded lever on the side of the boy's crib, Bailey and Meyerson recorded the frequency of lever pressing during a 7-day baseline period and found a mean of 135 responses per 24-hour day. Following this baseline period, vibration, produced by an apparatus mounted on the underside of the crib, was made contingent on lever pressing, such that each press produced 6 seconds of vibration. During the 21 days when this condition was in effect, the mean number of lever presses was more than 1,000, ranging from 700 to 2,000 per day. The responses were maintained on a steady rate for 3 weeks without decrement. When the vibration condition was discontinued, there was a striking decrease in lever pressing, with a drop to an average of 400 presses per day during the first week of this extinction phase.

When he was working the lever, the boy was observed to press the lever lightly with his hand or kick it with his foot and then to remain motionless or occasionally giggle while the vibrator was on. As soon as the vibration stopped, he would press the lever again. The data, together with this observation, indicate that this profoundly retarded boy had learned something and that the vibration was an effective reinforcer for lever pressing. While these authors do not report the relationship of the lever-pressing behavior to the self-stimulatory, injurious, stereotyped behavior the boy had displayed, it is possible that such behavior decreased while lever pressing was emitted at a high rate. Furthermore, as Bailey and

Meyerson point out, a simple behavior maintained with vibratory reinforcement might be considered a first step toward enlarging a child's repertoire to include more complex and useful forms of behavior.

Operant behavior modification technique has been applied with other retarded children to establish toilet training and such basic self-help skills as feeding and dressing. Giles and Wolf (1966), for example, through the use of positive reinforcers strengthened appropriate use of the toilet of five institutionalized, severely retarded males. This study points to the importance of finding suitable reinforcers for each child. While candy is an effective reinforcer for many children, Giles and Wolf found one boy who refused candy but accepted baby food; for others a ride in a wheelchair, taking a shower, or being permitted to return to bed were rewarding consequences. Giles and Wolf also point out that training can be improved if, in addition to the positive reinforcement of desired responses, inappropriate behavior is followed by aversive stimuli. Where positive reinforcement alone produced no results, they introduced physical restraint, the removal of which—contingent on appropriate toileting behavior—came to serve as a negative reinforcer. With this combination of techniques, all subjects learned consistently to eliminate in the toilet.

Roos and Oliver (1969) studied the effectiveness of operant-conditioning procedures using two control groups; one of which—a placebo group—received traditional special education training, while the other group received traditional institutional care. The results showed that the severely and profoundly retarded children in the experimental group made significantly greater progress in developing self-help skills than the two other groups. Beyond learning simple self-care skills, retarded children with IQ test scores as low as 30 have acquired appropriate classroom behavior (Birnbrauer, 1967), social skills (Baldwin, 1967), and academic subject matter (Birnbrauer, Bijou, Wolf, & Kidder, 1965).

The reason for referring to these studies is not to stress the effectiveness of operant procedures but to emphasize that the same principles of learning apply regardless of the degree of a child's retardation and that establishing this degree in terms of test scores becomes a very secondary matter, more useful for administrative-forensic than for therapeutic-educational purposes.

Since the consequences of a response are powerful factors in determining whether this response will be weakened or strengthened, those who wish to modify the behavior of retarded children—or of any children, for that matter—must, as we have said, first assess what conditions can serve as reinforcers. We are indebted to Zigler (1966a) for pointing to the differential effectiveness of reinforcers when retarded children, and particularly institutionalized retarded children, are compared with normal children, for this difference can account for many of the performance deficits of retarded children. In fact, the differences appear to be a function of institutionalization itself. In a series of studies Zigler (1966b) and his coworkers have shown that the effectiveness of social reinforcement is a function of the retardate's preinstitutional background. While the social deprivation which characterizes the institutional setting tends to make social reinforcement more potent for all institutional children, this effect is enhanced for those who come from relatively nondeprived homes as compared to those from more socially deprived backgrounds. In the long run, institutionalization is more socially depriving for children from good than for children from poor backgrounds, and follow-up studies (Zigler & Williams, 1963 ; Zigler, Butterfield, & Capobianco, 1970) demonstrate a decrease in social-reinforcer effectiveness that is greater for those with deprived preinstitutional histories. It thus appears that children from better backgrounds continue to be motivated by attention, praise, affection, and other social reinforcers, while for those from poorer backgrounds, these consequences gradually cease to be effective in maintaining behavior. When social reinforcers are ineffective, more tangible reinforcers, such as trinkets or food, can be used to reward behavior. Thus, Zigler and de Labry (1962), who found performance differences between normal and retarded children on a concept-switching task, demonstrated that when the consequences of success were changed to tangible rein-forcers, these differences disappeared. When an effective reinforcer is used, deficient performance can often be overcome—bearing out the contention that it is at least as important to assess what consti-tutes a reinforcing consequence for a given child as to count how many correct responses he can give on an intelligence test or to see what kind of a pattern his EEG tracings make on a piece of paper.

RECAPITULATION
Mental subnormality is a performance deficit which is associated with impairment in adaptive behavior. It is neither a disease entity nor necessarily a permanent, immutable state. There are a great many reasons why a given individual may be functioning at a subnormal level on tasks such as intelligence tests. Some children may be culturally disadvantaged, some developmentally retarded, and some limited in their potential. From the point of view of grouping mentally subnormal children it is helpful to speak of *familial retardation* and *organic retardation,* but in any specific case it is often difficult to determine the origin of the problem. Regardless of origin, all mentally subnormal children share a type of experience that has to do with their inability to meet the expectations of their social environment. These common experiences may be more important determinants of the behavior of these children than is the original cause of their subnormality. Approaches to the training of subnormal children that ignore the question of etiology and focus instead on the behavioral assets and deficits of the child and address these in a systematic fashion have been singularly successful.

7

JUVENILE DELINQUENCY

Juvenile delinquency is not a psychological term. It is a label the judicial system of society applies to children and adolescents who engage in behavior that the statutes define as illegal. Such behavior may range from curfew violation and loitering to theft, arson, and assault. It should therefore be obvious that the term *juvenile delinquent* designates a widely heterogeneous group of offenders so that any statement purporting to apply to all members of this group must be such a gross overgeneralization as to be meaningless.

The label juvenile delinquency covers a vast range of norm-violating behaviors, but it is applied to only a segment of those individuals who actually engage in such behavior. Technically, a person does not become a juvenile delinquent until so adjudged in court. Between the performance of the delinquent act and this adjudication there operates a selective process that results in the labeling of only an unknown proportion of the actual offenders as juvenile delinquents. This selection process is based not so much on the behavior of the youthful offender as on the behavior of others in relation to him and his offense. Someone must, first of all, discover the offense and bring the offender to the attention of an appropriate authority. If an individual police officer is involved, he may decide to limit his intervention to a stern reprimand, to send the youngster home, or to take him to the police station. Only some of those taken to the station are actually "booked," and not all whose act is thus recorded are then referred to the court. A variety of options are available to the court, ranging from an informal hearing, warning, and release to the parents, to probation, adjudication, parole, and commitment. Only the case that has been adjudicated delinquent enters official statistics on delinquency. Thus, data based on these statistics grossly distort any conclusions regarding incidence or prevalence. This is particularly true as far as conclusions regarding social class, neighborhoods, or ethnic background are concerned inasmuch as the various decisions made by the policeman and others regarding the disposition of the offender are influenced far more by who he is than by what he has done. When one attempts to gather delinquency statistics not from arrest records or court statistics but from anonymous self-reports of high school students (Nye, Short, & Olson, 1958), it emerges that norm-violating behavior has relatively little relationship to socioeconomic class.

DEFICIENT BEHAVIORAL CONTROLS

The norm violations committed by juvenile delinquents rarely involve complex skills that would have to be learned before the act could take place. Unlike such adult crimes as forgery, counterfeiting, or safecracking, most juvenile offenses, such as shoplifting, vandalism, or auto theft do not require a delinquency-specific skill. (Driving an automobile is a general skill; stealing a car with keys in the dashboard represents the application of this skill under unauthorized circumstances.) From this point of view it seems incorrect to speak of delinquency as learned behavior; it seems more productive to conceive of delinquency as behavior that reflects the offender's *failure to have learned* essential controls that most others in his society have acquired in the course of growing up. Most children learn what is and what is not acceptable behavior, and most acquire controls over their own behavior that keeps them from engaging in the unacceptable. The juvenile delinquent would thus be one who has either not learned to discriminate between accept-able and unacceptable behavior or who, having learned the discrimi-nation, has not acquired adequate controls so that his behavior is not guided by this discrimination. This formulation places the emphasis in a study of delinquency on deficient discrimination or deficient behavioral controls, and the prevention and treatment of delinquency would therefore have to focus on these deficiencies. It is this rea-soning which led to placing this chapter under the general rubric of *deficient behavior*.

Delay of Gratification

It is not unreasonable to assume that such delinquency-incompatible behaviors as remaining in school, holding a job, saving one's earnings, and similar norm-abiding acts require that one be able to maintain a response under conditions of delayed reinforcement. Delinquent behavior can thus be viewed as partly a function of an absence or weakness in the ability to delay gratification, to inhibit behavior for the sake of later reinforcement. The ability to defer gratification has been found to relate positively to a laboratory index of resistance to temptation (Mischel & Gilligan, 1964) and to ques-tionnaire data on social responsibility (Mischel, 1961).

Roberts and Erikson (1968) explored the relationship between measures of delay of gratification and ratings of adjustment in a school for delinquent adolescent males. A group of fifty subjects were asked to write an essay in answer to the following instruction: "A boy won $1,000 as first prize in a contest. What do you think he will do with it?" The responses were scored for delay of gratification on the basis of whether the boy saved the money or spent it imme-diately. Nine days before the subjects were scheduled for discharge, they were presented with a coupon which gave them the option of trading it for one cigarette or of holding it until their discharge at which point the coupon would be worth one package of cigarettes. The study revealed that those boys who were able to delay gratifica-tion on both the verbal (essay) and the behavioral measure received higher adjustment ratings from their supervisors. Since the subjects were already delinquents at the time this study was undertaken, it does not, of course, answer the question whether low impulse control led to the boys' delinquency in the first place. On the other hand, since the institutional supervisors can be viewed as representative of the norm-setting segment of society, their ratings suggest that the youngster who can delay gratification is more likely to be considered the "good guy" who obeys the rules and regulations than his impulsive peer who tends to be judged a "general nuisance."

The ability to delay gratification is acquired during childhood and can be shown to increase with age (Mischel & Metzner, 1962). In fact, one of the defining characteristics of social maturity is the ability to function under conditions of delayed reinforcement. The conditions under which this ability is acquired are not fully known, but laboratory studies suggest that opportunity to observe a model forgo immediate gratification for the sake of greater gratification later on is one means of inducing a child to behave similarly. Bandura and Mischel (1965), Mischel (1966), and Liebert and Ora (1968), have conducted a series of experiments in which a child is given the opportunity to observe another child or an adult who, given a choice between a small prize that can be obtained immediately and a larger prize for which one has to wait, selects the latter. When the observing child is later placed in a similar choice situation, he, too, will select the delayed reward even if the delay is for as much as 6 weeks.

Self-imposed Standards

The temporal delay of gratification is one expression of self-control; the self-imposition of reward standards is another. In the course of socialization a child must acquire the ability to evaluate his own performance and to develop standards for the self-administration of praise and tangible reinforcements. Self-reward is often considered as one aspect of "resistance to temptation." In experimental self-reward situations (Liebert & Ora, 1968) the child has material rewards available to him, and to the extent that he adheres to a norm requiring that these be taken sparingly he is exercising self-control. Exposing a child to a model who exemplifies self-reward behavior has been demonstrated to be a potent means of teaching this form of self-control (Liebert, Hanratty, & Hill, 1969; Allen & Liebert, 1969a, 1969b; Mischel & Liebert, 1967).

One dimension affecting the effectiveness of vicarious learning of self-reward standards is the model's consistency. Parents who demand a stringent level of achievement standards of their child while displaying self-indulgence in their own behavior may be particularly ineffective models. The consequence of such discrepant training was studied by Mischel and Liebert (1966) who asked children to participate with an adult model in a bowling game which seemingly required skill but on which scores were experimentally controlled. A plentiful supply of tokens, which could be exchanged for prizes, was available to both the model and the child. In one experimental group the model rewarded herself only for high levels of performance but told the child to reward himself for lower achievements; in a second condition the model rewarded herself for low performance but let the child reward himself only for higher achievement; while in a third group the model rewarded herself for high performance and told the child to reward himself only for equally high achievement. Following these procedures, measures were taken of the child's self-reward criteria while performing the task in the absence of the model or any other social agent. Children who had been permitted to reward themselves for relatively low performances during training by a self-stringent model showed no conflict about rewarding themselves for mediocre performance in the model's absence, and they did so uniformly. Children who had been instructed to reward themselves for only high performance levels by a model who also exhibited adherence to this stringent standard subsequently maintained the high criterion when left to perform entirely alone. In contrast to these two groups, children who had stringency imposed upon them but observed the model behave self-indulgently did not behave in a consistent fashion. Approximately half of the children in this group continued to adhere to the more stringent standard on which they had been directly trained, while the other half adopted the more lenient standards which they had observed. This investigation strongly suggests the importance for effective socialization of consistency between direct instruction and the performance modeled by the socializing agent.

It thus appears that delay of gratification and the self-imposition of reward standards can be learned by the vicarious mode of observing a model. Other controls and other modes of learning are no doubt relevant to the study of norm-violating behavior, and a variety of investigators have approached this issue from several different points of view.

THE LEARNING OF NORM-ABIDING BEHAVIOR

The process by which a child acquires delinquency-incompatible, norm-abiding behaviors and behavioral controls is frequently called *moral development*. Morality can be viewed as behavior regulated by the goals and norms of the group in which an individual lives. Such regulation requires that the individual has accepted these goals and norms as his own, an acceptance usually construed as *internalization*. This construct has been extensively studied by Kohlberg (1964) who approaches it from the standpoint of moral judgment and finds remarkable consistency in the different types of statements about moral situations obtained from individuals at different levels of "moral thinking."

Kohlberg (1964) speaks of the *preconventional*, the *conventional*, and the *postconventional* levels. The first of these levels is occupied by children between ages four and ten who tend to state standards of behavior largely in terms of physical consequences, i.e., reward and punishment. At the conventional level, the individual states rules of behavior in terms of their value in maintaining the social order, while at the highest level moral principles are viewed as autonomous abstractions. Within each of these three levels, Kohlberg discerns two stages. Stage one of the preconventional level entails an orientation toward punishment and the superior power of authority figures, while stage two individuals conform to rules to obtain rewards. At stage one of the conventional level, moral statements are framed in terms of seeking social approval for conforming to stereotyped images of acceptable behavior, and at stage two individuals verbalize concepts of "doing one's duty" and "respect for authority"; one conforms to avoid censure and resultant guilt. At the postconventional, highest level of morality, stage one entails conformity in order to maintain the social contract, while at stage two individuals verbalized such universal ethical principles as "justice," "equality," and "human dignity."

Kohlberg (1964) ascertains the moral level of an individual by seeking answers to such questions as "Is it better to save the life of one important person or a lot of unimportant people?" and by classifying the answer in terms of his moral stages. His work thus involves moral judgment, rather than moral behavior. While judgment may well play a role in guiding behavior, the relationship between the verbal statements obtained by Kohlberg and the actual behavior of his respondents remains to be established (Hess, 1970). Of greater relevance to the topic under consideration is research in which actual behavior along "moral" lines can be observed, although such studies have the weakness of requiring extrapolation from often highly artificial laboratory situations to conditions found in the daily life of individuals.

A sophisticated instance of such studies is the work of Aronfreed and Reber (1965) who investigated internalized behavioral suppression—that crucial step in moral development which permits an individual to move from Kohlberg's preconventional to the conventional level. For purposes of their study, Aronfreed and Reber viewed internalization to have taken place when a behavior, originally acquired under the control of an external agent, can be reliably elicited in the absence of such an agent. The children in this study had the task of picking up one of two toys and describing its use to the experimenter. When they picked up the more attractive of two toys, they were punished (mild social disapproval), while mild approval was contingent on their picking up the less attractive object. After nine such training trials, the experimenter left the child alone with a pair of toys and monitored his behavior to assess "transgression," defined as picking up the more attractive toy. The experimental variable of greatest interest was the timing of punishment; one group having been reprimanded as they reached for the more attractive toy, the other after they had held it for a few moments. The results showed that transgression was effectively prevented by punishment, with punishment at initiation more potent than punishment upon completion of the proscribed act.

On the basis of a review of this and similar research, Hoffman (1970) concluded that moral development is a complex phenomenon which ultimately leads to behavioral conformity; perception of authority as rational; impulse inhibition; and consideration for others. He suggests that four processes which may take place simultaneously and independently interact to bring about socialization in the moral realm. The first of these processes, according to Hoffman, consists of experiences involving differential reinforcement through reward and punishment of specific acts defined as "good" or "bad" by the agents of socialization. The behavior thus learned will generalize to similar situations, and if the reinforcement contingencies remain essentially unchanged, the behavioral standards learned in childhood will be maintained throughout life. This form of behavior control has its locus in the external environment and does not involve any internalization. The second process postulated by Hoffman moves behavior control beyond the mere avoidance of punishment and involves the child's perception of rules and authority as no longer arbitrary but as objective and rational. Experiences with rational authority figures who give reasons or explanations for demands that the child change his behavior and opportunities for him to assume the role of authority (as in participation in decision making) appear important requisites for this process.

The third process postulated in Hoffman's (1970) formulation of moral development may well be the most crucial in establishing internal controls over behavior. It entails the formation of what is generally known as conscience, traditionally called *superego*. Norm-abiding behavior ultimately depends not merely on avoidance of externally imposed consequences but, more importantly, on the avoidance of noxious stimulation which has its source within the individual ("guilt"). It appears that this step requires experiences with important adults who use "love-withdrawal" (as opposed to "power assertion") as a technique of child rearing. Love-withdrawal techniques take the form of parents expressing disapproval for undesirable behavior by contingent removal of such social reinforcers as attention, company, verbal exchange, and other forms of social interaction. It is essentially a form of suspension from social reinforcement ("time out") or, if one prefers, from "love." Hoffman (1970) points out that love-withdrawal has a highly punitive quality since it entails the threat of abandonment or separation. Since the parent's absence is likely to have been associated with painful or noxious stimulation sometime in the child's previous history (as when an infant is hungry but the mother is not immediately available for feeding), one can speculate that love-withdrawal has stimulus qualities that elicit noxious arousal (anxiety). When the stimulus qualities, elicited by love-withdrawal, are repeatedly paired with undesirable behavior, it is feasible that these behaviors and the cues associated with the immediate antecedents of these behaviors ("impulses") come to elicit the noxious arousal state, which should then lead to avoidance of the undesirable behavior, even in the absence of the parental figure. It is this arousal state, elicited by violations of norms or by the antici- pation of such violations, that is usually referred to as guilt and seen as an important factor in maintaining norm-abiding behavior.

The fourth process of moral development postulated by Hoffman (1970) involves the individual's capacity to control his behavior by considering its effect on the experiences of others, particularly the potential victims of proscribed behavior. This capacity for "empathy" presumably has its antecedents in parental statements involving explanations of the effects of one's behavior on others. The capacity for empathy requires considerable abstract ability and represents a rather advanced state in the development of moral behavior.

TYPES AND SOURCES OF DELINQUENCY

Failure to adhere to the conduct codes of society so that proscribed behavior comes to be emitted may be related to the temporary lapse of poorly established learned controls, to the failure to have learned these controls, or to the fact that the behavioral norms a child has learned do not coincide with the norms of that segment of society which writes and enforces the rules. These three conditions under which delinquent behavior may be observed permit one to speak of three forms of delinquency: the *impulsive delinquent*, the *unsocial- ized delinquent*, and the *socially delinquent*.

The impulsive delinquent has learned that stealing is punishable behavior; but on occasion, sometimes only once in his entire youth, the attractiveness of a given object, combined with a stimulus con- figuration that provides opportunity and a low probability of being detected, overwhelms his controls so that the antisocial act is performed. As with any other behavior, its future course will be a function of its consequences. If they are negative—the child is caught and punished or he experiences subjective discomfort in anticipation of potential punishment (guilt)—the probability of repetition is lowered. If the consequences are positive—the child is not punished, he experiences minimal subjective discomfort, and the stolen object serves as a reinforcer—the probability is increased that the action will be repeated when similar circumstances again present themselves.

The unsocialized delinquent is an individual whose behavior has developed under conditions of learning that failed to establish the internal controls which keep most people in his culture from committing antisocial acts. It is a fair assumption that these conditions of learning are found in the child's family during his formative years, and several well-known studies (e.g., Glueck & Glueck, 1950, 1959, 1962; McCord & McCord, 1959) have focused on the family structure and parent-child relationship of juvenile delinquents. There is, of course, no one-to-one relationship between background variables and delinquency, and it is fallacious to assume that all delinquents have a common background or that background factors found with relatively high frequency among delinquents will differentiate delinquents from nondelinquents. Studies always show that a large percentage of delinquents have the background commonly found among nondelinquents and, conversely, that there are nondelinquents with backgrounds commonly found among delinquents. It is thus totally unwarranted to assume in any specific case of delinquency that a given set of family conditions were present. This point bears stressing because, as Cavan (1962) has observed, "A commonly held psychiatric view is that virtually all delinquency is an indication of early parental neglect or rejection" (p. 177).

Glueck and Glueck (1959) have identified a series of family factors which permit one to predict delinquent behavior with reasonable accuracy when one studies *groups* of children; for any *specific* child predictions are hazardous. The Glueck Social Prediction Table associates the following with potential delinquency: *overstrict or erratic paternal discipline, unsuitable maternal supervision, paternal indifference or hostility, maternal indifference or hostility, and lack of family cohesiveness (weak affectional ties and few shared interests).*

When these factors were assigned weighted scores based on the frequency with which they were found among a sample of delinquents, lack of family cohesiveness and maternal indifference or hostility to the boy were the most heavily weighted factors. While such a finding is highly suggestive, about one-third of a group of 890 delinquent and nondelinquent children fell in a midrange of scores where predictive validity is very low.

The Cambridge-Somerville Youth Study (Powers & Witmer, 1951) was a large-scale project in which 253 boys were intensively studied, and those among them who became delinquent were followed up 20 years later. When McCord and McCord (1959) evaluated the results of this work, they found that the environmental factors most likely to lead to delinquent behavior were a combination of absence of maternal warmth and a criminal paternal role model. Similarly, Bandura and Walters (1959) reported that the aggressive delinquent boys they had studied came from families marked by parental inconsistency in child rearing and rejection by fathers who used physically punitive methods of discipline.

The acquisition of behavior controls that seem weak or absent in the unsocialized delinquent would seem to require the following: consistency in the consequences parents bring to bear on the child's behavior; clear guidelines as to what is acceptable behavior; positively regarded, good role models; and conditions under which social approval can acquire secondary reinforcement potential. When these conditions are absent, the probability that a boy raised in such a family will come to be identified as a delinquent appears greatly increased.

Delinquency and Social Class

It has often been reported that there is a higher probability for delinquent behavior among lower-class than middle- or upper-class children (Short & Strodtbeck, 1965). This relationship holds for urban areas; but when urban and rural communities are compared (Clark & Wenninger, 1962; Erickson & Empey, 1965), it can be shown that delinquency rate is not a function of social class per se but of factors associated with social class, such as neighborhood, family structure, and peer associations. The environmental conditions in the urban lower-class neighborhood would seem to be more likely to favor the development of delinquent behavior than would the conditions found in other areas. Parental preoccupations with day-to-day survival questions, father absence, and limited family resources around which to develop shared interests may conspire to produce the conditions which were so predictive of delinquency in the Glueck and Glueck (1959) studies. It stands to reason that delinquency is a function of a complex interaction of factors and that any one condition—be it father absence, the "broken home," poverty, or erratic discipline—is not likely to be a direct cause.

One-parent households are found more frequently among delinquents than among nondelinquents. In comparing 500 delinquent boys with 500 nondelinquent boys, Glueck and Glueck (1950) found that 34.6 percent of the delinquent, but only 19.8 percent of the nondelinquent, lived with only one parent, usually the mother. Findings of this kind have led to theories about the role of the "female-based household" in the development of delinquency (Miller, 1958). Such a household may exist for a variety of reasons and have a great many implications in terms of the child's socialization. Absence of the father may be due to death, separation, desertion, or divorce. In each instance a good deal of interpersonal conflict or trauma may have preceded the actual time the father left the household, and assumptions about the effect of the "broken home" on the child must take these facts into consideration. Nye (1958), for example, has pointed out that broken but happy homes produce less delinquency than intact but unhappy homes. A second condition leading to a "female-based household" involves the absence from his birth onward of a legal or stable union between the child's mother and father. Since such a family does not represent a breakdown of a marriage but is often an accepted pattern in certain subcultures, there is no reason to assume that the child will have experienced conflict between father and mother or the trauma involved in a father's death or departure. At the same time poverty, social disintegration, lack of recreational and educational opportunities, and easy access to delinquent role models are often correlated with this subcultural family pattern, and so it is extremely difficult to ascertain which factor or combinations of factors contribute to delinquency.

Father absence is usually seen as representing the absence of the stricter disciplinarian and the lack of a masculine role model. While these generalizations may have some merit, one should not lose sight of other implications the one-parent home has for the child's socialization. Among these are the greater demands on the mother's time and energy which are likely to strain her relationship to the child. Her demands for compliance may increase, while, at the same time, her consistency in enforcing them may be low. In the two-parent household reinforcements are dispensed by both parents and when one parent is nonreinforcing because of preoccupation or anger at the child, the other parent may be available to provide succor. Under conditions of father absence, the peer group may early become an important source of reinforcements, social support, and role models.

The availability of unsupervised, unoccupied groups of same sex peers tends to be greater in the lower-class than in the middle-class neighborhood, giving rise to a class-related phenomenon of *gang delinquency* where the peer group, operating within its own value system, supports and reinforces the delinquent behavior of its members. It is here that the individual youngster may learn a set of behavioral norms that are approved by those who are important sources of reinforcement for him but that happen to run counter to the norms of behavior approved and enforced by the modal group in society. Such an individual may acquire controls over his own behavior, but these controls tend to lead him to conform to the delinquent standards of his social reference group; hence the term *socially delinquent* is sometimes used to describe this type.

Conditions of learning in the lower-class culture   The norms, values, and "focal concerns" of the lower-class culture have been discussed by Miller (1958) who sees them as the generating milieu of gang delinquency. The observations of this cultural anthropologist are based on extensive work by seven trained social workers who maintained contact with twenty-one street-corner groups in a slum district for a period of 3 years. Miller lists, roughly in order of importance, six focal concerns (values) of people in the lower-class culture. They are trouble, toughness, smartness, excitement, fate, and autonomy. Since the reinforcement contingencies of the lower-class peer group are largely guided by these focal concerns which thus represent important conditions of social learning for each of its members, these focal concerns bear some elaboration.

TROUBLE   Getting into and staying out of trouble is a dominant feature of lower-class culture, and the alternatives are generally between "law-abiding" and "non-law-abiding" behavior. According to Miller (1958) individuals are judged in relation to these behavioral alternatives, and status is gauged along this dimension. Thus, a mother will assess the suitability of a given boy as a companion for her daughter less on the basis of his achievement potential, as she would in the middle class, but on the basis of his likelihood of getting into trouble. With limited opportunities for skill attainment and educational achievement, "getting into trouble" is one of the few ways by which an individual can obtain attention and recognition from his peers; hence behavior that is likely to get one into trouble may be reinforced. In fact, as Miller points out, in certain situations, "getting into trouble" is a source of prestige, and some adolescent groups (gangs) make membership contingent on a demonstration of law-violating behavior.

TOUGHNESS   This concern has its focus on behaviors that are considered signs of "masculinity" such as physical prowess, bravery in the face of physical threat, lack of sentimentality, and an exploitative attitude toward women. Some of these qualities, such as strength and endurance, have a good deal of survival value in a street-corner culture of the inner city; others are modeled and reinforced by the peer group as conforming to the defined masculine role. Behavior which is incompatible with that role, including interest in the literature or art of the middle class, or "soft" and sentimental behavior, elicits negative reactions from the peer group, which evaluates such behavior as role-inappropriate and derides it with terms associated with homosexuality such as "fag" or "queer."

SMARTNESS   In this focal concern, value is placed on the ability to attain a goal, such as material goods or personal status, through mental agility. It involves the ability to outwit, outsmart, and outfox others while avoiding having others "take," "con," or dupe you. The peer group not only provides the training ground for this ability through mutual teasing, kidding, razzing, and "ranking" but it also rewards smartness by assigning leadership roles and high prestige to the individual with demonstrated skill in this area. Miller (1958) points out that the street-corner group allocates leadership roles to both the tough and the smart with the ideal leader combining both capacities. In a choice between smartness and toughness, the former tends to be the more prestigious quality—reflecting, according to Miller, a general lower-class respect for "brain" in the sense of shrewdness, wit, and adroitness in verbal repartee.

EXCITEMENT   Like the other focal concerns of the lower-class culture, this one represents a bipolar continuum ranging from thrill to boredom. Life fluctuates between these extremes with brief periods of thrill and emotional stimulation alternating with longer periods of boredom and routine. Excitement—involving elements of risk and danger—is actively sought and accompanied by use of alcohol, gambling, sexual adventuring, and music. Fights are not infrequent aspects of excitement in view of this volatile mixture of activities. The breaks in routine characterizing excitement clearly involve the "focal concerns" previously mentioned, since toughness and smartness are brought into play and trouble frequently follows.

FATE   Largely as a function of the conditions under which he is raised and lives, the lower-class individual tends to view the locus of control over his life as outside himself. A set of poorly comprehended forces over which he has relatively little control tend to determine the lower-class individual's experiences. Positive experiences are thus attributed to fate, luck, or fortune, while negative events are similarly explained as a function of unlucky destiny. Miller (1958) points out that the pervasive gambling in the lower class is a reflection of this orientation, though gambling also involves smartness and excitement.

AUTONOMY   This involves a concern with independence and freedom from external constraints or superordinate authority. Concern with autonomy finds expression in such statements as "No one's gonna push *me* around" or "I don't need *nobody* to take care of me." Again it interrelates with other concerns, such as smartness, toughness, and trouble. Since getting into trouble often entails an encounter with restrictive, superordinate authority, there is a certain incompatibility of these two values, and a good deal of excitement can ensure when one has to use one's smartness to flirt with trouble and yet preserve one's autonomy.

We have mentioned in passing that the male adolescent peer group in lower-class society supports these focal concerns by making status and group membership contingent on the individual's adherence to these values. In Miller's (1958) formulation *belonging* and *status* become focal concerns specific to the street-corner group, but these are on a higher level of abstraction than the six concerns previously discussed inasmuch as they are the means by which belonging and status are attained.

At this point it may be well to examine the implications of the focal concerns identified by Miller in terms of their possible contribution to delinquent behavior. If the peer group is an important, and, in some cases, an almost exclusive source of reinforcement, the values of this group will importantly shape the individual's behavior. It is apparent that the focal concerns of the lower-class ethos as postulated by Miller (1958) not only favor adolescent behavior that society-at-large has defined as delinquent but in many respects they also are incompatible with such norm-abiding activities as working or going to school which, were they engaged in, might provide the adolescent with an alternate source of reinforcement. If freedom from constraint, outwitting the other, physical prowess, skirting trouble with the law, and a reliance on luck instead of personal initiative and effort are the means of maintaining group membership and status, one is far more likely to engage in theft, assault, or destruction of property than to seek and hold gainful employment. These value-based behavioral tendencies interact with the social and economic conditions in which the lower-class child grows up. As Cloward and Ohlin (1960) have pointed out, it is far more likely that an individual seeks gratification through illegitimate means when the accessibility of gratification through legitimate means is limited or closed altogether. In an environment of this kind, the adolescent lacks access to adults who might present role models for socially constructive behavior; he has available to him models of socially disapproved behavior, and he fails to develop the skills necessary for success in society-at-large and by the means this society approves. It is this lack of skills, not only the academic skills taught in school but also such social skills as making a favorable impression in a job interview and coming to work regularly and on time, that become major blocks to success within the approved norms.

The role of parents   In laboratory experiments it can be shown that the most effective means of teaching suppression of a response is to introduce punishment at the *initiation* of the act (Mowrer & Aiken, 1954; Walters & Demkow, 1963). In their theoretical analysis of learned behavior suppression Aronfreed and Reber (1965) address themselves to the question why, despite the importance of the timing of punishment demonstrated in such experiments, self-control can be acquired in the course of naturalistic socialization where the negative consequences of transgression rarely coincide with response initiation.

Among the features of the naturalistic setting which Aronfreed and Reber (1965) identify as possibly diluting the significance of timing is the strong positive attachment of a child to his parents. With that, parental disapproval, no matter when expressed in relation to the time of transgression, may elicit far greater intensity of anxiety than can be aroused by an experimenter in the laboratory. Greater intensity of anxiety would result in a raising of the generalization gradient, and so it could motivate suppression at the point of incipient transgression, even though punishment was originally dispensed at a later point in time. It is also true, as Aronfreed and Reber point out, that parents who maintain reasonably close surveillance over their child's behavior will have occasion to dispense punishment in the form of disapproval or verbal warning while a transgression is taking place, thus moving punishment closer to the point of initiation and increasing its effectiveness. Furthermore, parents, who are effective in helping their child establish internal behavior controls, will frequently be aware of evidence of response suppression in their child's behavior and reinforce such instances of self-control with affection, praise, or other reward. Lastly, but most important in terms of the context of this discussion, Aronfreed and Reber (1965) stress the role of language in the development of self-control. They state that the most effective feature in insuring internalized suppression, regardless of the temporal locus of punishment in the transgression sequence, is the extensive verbalization with which parents point out the nature of the child's transgression, the events preceding their occurrence, and the negative consequences for both the child and other people. This technique of *induction* (Hoffman, 1970) makes it possible for conceptual labeling and other cognitive processes to arouse anxiety around incipient transgressions so that suppression of the transgression can become negatively reinforced by anxiety reduction. Verbal communication between parent and child also enables the child to recognize and associate with anxiety, intentions and other antecedents of a committed transgression so that on future occasions anxiety will be elicited by these cognitive representations themselves.

Many of the features that would contribute to the establishment of internal behavior controls, such as close parental surveillance, love-oriented child-rearing practices, and the use of induction, may be more frequently found in the middle-class than in the lower-class family. Middle-class parents, say Aronfreed and Reber (1965), are more oriented toward their children's intentions, more likely to resort to reasoning and explanation in hopes of establishing internal controls, and more active in inducing their children to initiate their own self-corrective processes. Lower-class parents, in contrast, are more likely to react to the concrete consequences of child transgression and to use aversive controls, so-called "power assertion" (Hoffman, 1970), when transgressions come to their attention. Punishment is more direct and less frequently accompanied by explanatory verbalizations. Aronfreed and Reber also believe that lower-class parents are less likely than middle-class parents to reinforce instances of response suppression.

The research support for the postulated social-class differences in the establishment of internal controls is somewhat indirect, making the statements of Aronfreed and Reber challenging hypotheses rather than established fact. Kohlberg (1963), for example, reports social-class differences in maturity of moral judgment, but research by Boehm and Nass (1962) shows that these differences may be a function of differences in level of intellectual development. On the other hand, there is reasonably strong support, particularly from the studies by Hess and Shipman (1965, 1967), for the statements regarding social-class differences in linguistic modes in mother-child interaction.

Reinforcement Contingencies

While studies on delinquent youths identify social class as an important variable in the development of norm-violating behavior (Short, 1966), the relationship among lower-class child-rearing methods, linguistic patterns, moral judgment, internal controls, and delinquent behavior is far too tenuous to permit causal generalizations beyond the truism that a child's early environment will have an impact on his later behavior, including behavior judged delinquent. The important contributions made to the development and maintenance of delinquent behavior by environmental, social-learning factors are highlighted by Schwitzgebel (1964, 1967) whose pioneering studies approached delinquency from the point of view of a functional analysis of behavior. Such an analysis seeks to establish what conditions maintain a given behavior so that, by modifying the conditions, the behavior can be changed. Further, and more importantly however, a functional analysis of behavior specifies the desired end point of behavior change as concretely as possible and identifies the behavioral steps necessary for reaching this end point. By assessing a given individual's behavior repertoire, one can then determine what the individual has to learn in order to move him toward the desired criterion behavior.

Schwitzgebel (1964) worked with 30 white males with a mean age of 18 years who had been adjudged delinquent by the courts, 20 of them having spent 6 months or more in correctional institutions. Through successive approximations and positive reinforcement these young men were taught such employment-compatible social skills as coming to work on time, being dressed appropriately, and limiting hostile statements in their conversation. In addition, they were taught to solder and other similar technical skills before they were helped to find jobs in the community. On follow-up 3 years later the arrest and incarceration record of the first 20 subjects was about half of that of a matched control group whose names had been obtained from police records. The effectiveness of this skill-centered social-learning approach stands in marked contrast to the disappointing results of earlier attempts at delinquency prevention which usually focused counseling and psychotherapeutic efforts on the subjects' presumed "character structure" and "inner conflicts" (McCord & McCord, 1959; Toby, 1965).

One of the investigations conducted by Schwitzgebel (1967) within the confines of the larger project dealt with the differential effectiveness of positive reinforcement (praise, cigarettes, candy, etc.) and mild punishment (interviewer's inattention and mild verbal disagreement). He reports that the positive consequences were effective in increasing positive statements, but that the negative consequences failed to decrease hostile statements. While this is in no way a conclusive test of the effectiveness of punishment, a study by Schlichter and Ratliff (1971) lends support to the conclusion that punishment is not as effective a means of facilitating learning in delinquents as it is with nondelinquents. These investigators matched

45 delinquent males committed to a correctional institution with an equal number of students from a junior high school who had no record of delinquency. These subjects were observed in a two-choice discrimination task with either positive reinforcement for correct responses or punishment for incorrect responses, or a combination of both positive reinforcement for correct responses and punishment for incorrect responses, respectively. Reinforcement consisted of poker chips which could be exchanged for money; the punishment was a loud (98-decibel) tone which signified that the subject was "losing" on what was presented as a "learning problem." The results showed that the nondelinquents performed better in the punishment condition than did the delinquents, whereas the delinquents performed better in the reward condition than the nondelinquents. Further, for the nondelinquent group the punishment condition was significantly more effective than the reward condition in producing correct responses.

Before one erroneously concludes from the studies of Schwitzgebel (1967) and of Schlichter and Ratliff (1971) that delinquents become such because they are less responsive than normals to punishment and social disapproval, it is well to recall that these data were gathered *after* these young people had been labeled delinquent and, in most instances, had spent time in correctional institutions. It is therefore important to ask what possible effect these circumstances might have on the individual's performance under the conditions of (mild) punishment used in these studies. Schlichter and Ratliff (1971) conjecture about the effects of the probable reinforcement histories with authority figures of delinquents and nondelinquents. They assume that the experimenter was regarded as an authority figure since he was working with the approval of the people in charge of the institutions. They further assume "that delinquents have experienced fewer positive reinforcements and nondelinquents, fewer punishments from authorities"; therefore

it follows that positive reinforcement for delinquents and punishment for normals may represent unusual events which are contrary to their expectancies and, therefore, serve to heighten attention to the task itself. Such heightened attention should serve to facilitate performance for delinquents in the reward condition and performance for nondelinquents in the punishment condition [p. 48].

Regardless of whether or not these speculations are correct, it stands to reason that one cannot assume a priori that any given consequence for behavior will have an effect with any given individual, be he delinquent or nondelinquent. As was done in the Schwitzgebel (1967) study, the effectiveness of a given consequence, be it reward or punishment, must be ascertained for each and every individual whom one wishes to teach a new response. In that respect a generalized reinforcer, such as a token or money which can be exchanged for an object of high valence for the individual, clearly has a greater chance of being effective than a uniform consequence like a 98-decibel noise. The effectiveness of behavior-modification programs for juvenile delinquents, such as those described by Burchard and Tyler (1965), Staats and Butterfield (1965), Tharp and Wetzel (1969), and Tyler and Brown (1968), seems largely a function of the systematic and response-contingent use of potent consequences.

RECAPITULATION

The norm-violating behavior society labels *delinquent* can be construed as a function of deficient behavioral controls. Among these are the ability to respond under conditions of delayed reinforcement (delay of gratification) and the self-imposition of standards (resistance to temptation). These behavioral controls and delinquency-incompatible, norm-abiding behavior are learned, and the study of delinquency must therefore turn to a study of the conditions under which such learning takes place and fails to take place. Important among these conditions are experiences with differential reinforcement of acceptable and unacceptable behavior, encounters with rational authority figures, the establishment of internal controls, and the capacity to consider the effects of one's behavior on others. For many reasons, the circumstances conducive to these conditions are often absent in the lower-class culture where the value system tends to be incompatible with the norms imposed by the middle class. When rehabilitation programs focus on important social and occupational skills, long-standing patterns of delinquent behavior can often be reversed.

8

PSYCHOPHYSIOLOGICAL DISORDERS

In our discussion of determinants of behavior, found in Chapter 1, we pointed out that any specific behavior, taking place at any one point in time, represents the end point of the interaction of an individual's genetic-constitutional factors, his past learning, his current physiological state, and his current environmental conditions. In some psychological disorders the interaction between environmental conditions and the physiological state is more obvious than in others—the responses prominently involving those factors conventionally called *psychological* and those considered *physiological.* This is the case in asthma, certain eating and elimination difficulties, skin disorders, ulcers of the gastrointestinal tract, and similar problems involving the body and its functions. For a discussion of difficulties in this area the term *psychophysiological disorders* is a convenient chapter heading, but the use of this term, or the exclusion of other disorders from this chapter, should not lead one to forget that physiological conditions play a role in every form of human behavior, hence, in every behavior disorder.

Traditionally, the disorders discussed in this chapter were called *psychosomatic disorders,* a term we prefer to avoid because it has come to carry the unwarranted connotation that in these disorders psychological factors "cause" the bodily (somatic) reactions. For example, in a chapter headed "Mind and Body," Kessler (1966) discusses "emotional causes for somatic symptoms" and reviews the simplistic formulations which would attribute the cause of a given physiological disorder (say, asthma) to a specific aspect of the child's experience (maternal rejection). The formulation according to which there is a directional causality from the psychological to the physiological is an anachronistic relic of the once-popular mind-body dualism that René Descartes advanced in the 17th Century in order to prove the existence of the human soul.

In a scholarly review of psychophysiological disorders of children Lipton, Steinschneider, and Richmond (1966) report that they failed to "discern specific psychological conflicts in specific diseases" (p. 212) and point instead to a complex interaction of individually differentiated constitutional predispositions and environmental situations. While this hypothesis of interaction has appeal, the research support for it is largely indirect since the very complexity of the formulation calls for highly complex, sophisticated studies that, by and large, remain to be carried out. Such studies will undoubtedly be facilitated if it is recognized that such gross categories as *asthma* for all children with expiratory distress, *anorexia nervosa* for all who refuse to eat, or *eczema* for a great variety of skin disorders may each subsume different disorders which one studies in undifferentiated groups at the cost of obfuscation.

It has been demonstrated (Richmond & Lustman, 1955) that there are marked individual differences in autonomic functions within the first days of life. Neonates differ in changes of skin temperature and heart rate in response to a variety of stimuli, and these differences follow a normal distribution with hyperreactors at one extreme and hyporeactors at the other. When such constitutional deviations from the norm interact with a given combination of environmental events, among which maternal behavior no doubt plays a major role, it is likely that a psychophysiological disorder can develop. On the other hand, a child with atypical autonomic reactions who encounters a different set of environmental events might well go through life without developing such a disorder.

This interactional formulation attributes the cause of psychophysiological disorders neither to purely biological nor to purely environmental factors. The complex development of such a disorder is next to impossible to analyze into its component interacting factors when an individual child with a psychophysiological problem is studied after he has lived with this disorder for a number of years. Like any child with a persistent health problem which began in early childhood, his problem will have complicated his relationship to his parents and particularly to his mother whose caretaking efforts will have been affected. Like children with chronic diseases the child may well have developed atypical dependency on his mother, but theories which view this dependency as the cause rather than the effect of the disorder are not well founded.

ASTHMA

The physical symptoms of asthma are difficulty in inspiring and, particularly, expiring air. This is accompanied by sensations of chest tightening and a characteristic wheezing during the expiratory phase of breathing. These symptoms are observed in a variety of conditions, including so-called asthmatic bronchitis and some allergies, not all of which are appropriately classified as asthma (Lipton et al., 1966). It has been proposed (Turnbull, 1962) that asthma is a learned response, but while the onset of asthmatic attack appears related to social situations, it remains to be demonstrated that differential reinforcement can establish asthma in a child who does not have a constitutional predisposition.

Because many clinical observations have pointed to the parent-child relationship as an important factor in precipitating asthmatic attacks, Purcell and his associates (1969) conducted a crucial study designed to assess the effect of experimentally separating the child from his family. In the past, such separations usually involved moving the child from his home. However this separation confounds the experiment because the child is also removed from potential allergic agents in the home, such as dust, pollens, or animal fur, which leaves unanswered the question whether asthmatic attacks are due to psychosocial or allergic factors, or both. In addition to separating these two factors, the Purcell study also throws light on the question whether asthmatic attacks are associated with impending or threatened separation from the mother (since some have speculated that the "wheeze" is a distorted cry for the mother). The study also supports the contention that asthmatic children do not form one homogeneous group but that there are subgroups among these children for whom a variety of stimuli serve as trigger for asthmatic attacks.

The subjects in the Purcell study were twenty-five asthmatic children with a mean age of 8 years, 4 months. On the basis of detailed interviews the group was divided into those whose asthmatic attacks were usually preceded by emotional arousal, such as anger, anxiety, excitement, or sadness. There were thirteen such children. The other twelve had a history of asthmatic attacks that did not appear to be precipitated by emotional arousal. On the basis of earlier work (Purcell, 1963) the investigators predicted that separation from the family would result in improvement for the asthmatic children with emotional precipitants, while the others would show no change.

Two of the measures used to assess change—expiratory peak flow rate (gauging the speed with which the child is able to expel air) and scaled degree of wheezing—were taken during daily laboratory visits; the other two—daily medications and daily history of asthma—were based on reports from the adult caretaker. The investigators took the base-rate measures while the child was at home with his family and during a period when impending separation was explicitly discussed. The family then moved out of the home, and the child stayed there with a carefully selected substitute mother. The separation lasted 2 weeks after which the family returned. The measures were collected during the entire time the family was absent, upon reunion, and into the post-reunion period. Figure 7 shows the data for the expiratory peak flow rate for the 13 children with emotional precipitants.

Contrary to the speculation that asthma is related to fear of separation from the mother, there was no increase on any of the measures during the pre-separation period. Furthermore, and in confirmation of the investigators' predictions, the experimental separation resulted in improvement on all four measures for the thirteen children

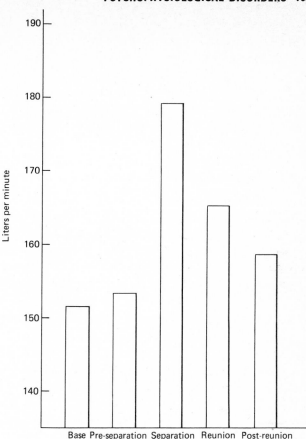

Periods

Fig. 7. Mean daily expiratory peak flow rate for thirteen asthmatic children with emotional precipitants. (After Purcell et al., 1969.) Copyright 1969 by the American Psychosomatic Society and reproduced by permission.

whose asthma appeared emotion-related. Only one measure (daily asthma) reflected improvement for the other twelve children, suggesting that even for these, psychosocial factors played some role in precipitating attacks. Using a rather stringent criterion of improvement for each individual child (as opposed to improvement on group-based measures), Purcell reports that during the period of separation seven of the thirteen emotion-related cases improved, while only three of the twelve for whom no improvement had been predicted showed a positive change. One of the most interesting aspects of this carefully conducted study is that following reunion with their families, all measures for all children returned to the base-rate, pre-separation level. This strongly suggests that asthmatic attacks are under the control of stimuli associated with family members, but these results cannot be used to support an argument that psychosocial factors alone were originally responsible for the child's asthma.

A speculation based on the interaction hypothesis would lead one to assume that some children have a constitutional tendency for an atypical respiratory pattern and that this comes to interact with environmental conditions following the operant paradigm. The principles of operant learning require that a response must be emitted before it can come under control of environmental stimuli. The higher the operant rate of a response (that is, its "natural" rate before conditioning has taken place), the higher the probability that the response will be emitted in the presence of a given set of circumstances that can come to serve as discriminative and reinforcing stimuli. Since breathing is one of the most frequently occurring responses and inasmuch as changes in rate of breathing are reflexive reactions to sudden changes in stimulation, it would not be unexpected that for children with an atypical breathing pattern, maternal behavior can come to be associated with respiratory distress, since such behavior would have countless opportunities to become contingent on respiratory responses of the child.

OBESITY AND FOOD REFUSAL

Eating is another response that, while not as frequent as breathing, takes place so many times in a child's early life that it would be surprising if the mother's behavior did not become an important discriminative and reinforcing stimulus. During the first few years of life, the presence of the mothering person is, in fact, an inevitable discriminative stimulus for food intake. In addition, food intake, after a period of relative food deprivation, represents a positive consequence for eating behavior, and so the behavior carries its own, inherent reinforcer. This combination of circumstances, the reinforcing nature of eating and—at least in the early years—the inevitable presence of the mother while eating takes place, makes this situation a potent setting for learning.

Obesity, the physical state of overweight, is usually the result of overeating, although in some instances it may involve a metabolic disorder. It is not clear to what extent a constitutional predisposition plays a role in obesity; the fact that many obese children have obese parents can be explained, as we shall see, without recourse to genetic speculations. Like so many other psychological disorders, obesity is a relative concept. Except in extreme instances, the point at which a chubby, sturdy child should be considered "overweight" depends on his deviation from the age-height-weight norm for his sex in his society. Some investigators (e.g., Bruch, 1961) use an arbitrary cutoff point whereby a child's weight must be 25 percent above the norm before he is classified as obese.

Food intake is positively reinforcing only to the point of satiation; beyond this, further eating becomes aversive and will be avoided unless powerful reinforcers are operating which, on balance, are stronger than the avoidance tendencies. In the case of the obese child, one must look for these postulated reinforcers in order to ascertain what maintains his overeating. In the absence of systematic research on this topic, clinical observations suggest that among the reinforcing conditions for excessive eating are the behavior of an oversolicitous mother who rewards the child's eating by offering extrinsic reinforcers, possibly because watching her child eat has reinforcing implications for her. It is also possible that feelings of comfort, associated with the feeding period in the child's early years, have acquired secondary reinforcement value and serve to maintain eating behavior beyond the point of satiation, particularly when the child has limited alternate sources of comfort. One also observes that obese children often have one or two obese parents, leading to the speculation that these parents model or reward excessive eating or both. In some cases overeating may be maintained by negative reinforcement, since obesity permits a child to avoid peer competition in physical activity and sports or in social interaction such as attending dances, skating parties, hikes and the like, any or all of which may be aversive to a given child. It is unlikely that the overeating was originally learned through avoidance conditioning (a child does not begin to overeat "in order to" have a reason for not joining the track team), but once learned, the behavior may well be maintained in this manner.

Food refusal, the logical opposite of overeating, is traditionally known as anorexia nervosa, "nervous loss of appetite." The objective result of food refusal is loss of weight, and the definition of this problem usually includes a reference to excessive weight loss. Some (e.g., Bliss & Branch, 1960) define excessive weight loss in terms of absolute pounds, although setting the cutoff point in terms of a percentage would be a more useful criterion, particularly in the case of children. With the definitional emphasis placed on weight loss, this category also includes persistent vomiting following feeding, which can be viewed as a variant of food refusal. This discussion of excessive weight loss through food refusal or persistent vomiting is, of course, limited to instances where it is clearly a psychological problem and not the result of physical illness.

Clinical histories of children who display food refusal often include parents for whom food has some special significance, either in terms of their overeating or in their need to maintain a diet for medical reasons. As might be expected, eating or not eating has long played a role in such a child's interaction with his parents, and many of these children have had periods of excessive food intake before they finally come to clinical attention because of the weight loss. Of interest is the fact that food refusal is one of the few disorders which have a higher frequency among girls than boys, some investigators (Bliss & Branch, 1960) reporting a ratio as high as 9 to 1. Another characteristic feature is that these underweight, often emaciated, children and adolescents emit verbalizations to the effect that they are not too thin, some, in fact, insisting that they are too fat (Blitzer et al., 1961).

There are probably a variety of developmental events and environmental conditions that will lead to the end state recognized as food refusal. One formulation, proposed by Bruch (1961, 1962), suggests that individuals have to learn appropriate labels for various bodily sensations and that these labels then come to guide behavior that is relevant to these sensations. According to this, a child would have to learn the label *hunger* for the sensations related to food deprivation, and having learned this label, he could learn to engage in food-seeking behavior when he recognizes the sensation. While this formulation has a distinctly counterintuitive quality (food-seeking when hungry seems such a "natural" response), research supporting attribution theory (Schachter & Singer, 1962; Valins, 1967) lends some credence to this view. Attribution theory holds that people attribute their internal sensations to external stimuli; that is, they "explain" how they feel by circumstances under which the feeling is experienced. The theory further states that social influences and the learning of labels importantly affect a person's attributions (Nisbett & Valins, 1971). If some children fail to learn correctly to label the sensations accompanying nutritional need, they might literally not know when they are hungry and when they are sated. Reports that many anorexic children have gone through earlier periods of excessive eating would be consonant with this speculation. Another source of indirect support is the fact that food refusal is largely an adolescent phenomenon. Until adolescence, food intake tends to be controlled by the mother; the child does not have to know when to eat and when not to eat. With the increasing independence from maternal control which comes with adolescence, however, the individual who does not seek food when he is objectively hungry because he mislabels the subjective sensation would lose weight rather precipitously. When the mother then steps back into the picture, urging the adolescent to eat, conflict over control and independence may well complicate the problem. It must, of course, also be remembered that adolescence is a period of drastic changes in the biochemistry of the body and of great changes in body build, factors which have led some to attribute adolescent eating problems either to biochemical dysfunction (Anand, 1961) or to conflicts about becoming a woman (Bliss & Branch, 1960).

Treatment Approaches

While the efficacy of a given method of treatment does not throw light on the etiology of the disorder so treated, a careful analysis of the variables operating in the treatment approach does reveal some of the factors currently maintaining the disorder. One such analysis was reported by Leitenberg, Agras, and Thomson (1968) who treated two adolescent girls who manifested food refusal. Both complained of "lack of appetite," frequently vomited after eating, expressed fear of obesity, and had menstrual disturbances (amenorrhea), a frequent concomitant of anorexia. The first case, a fourteen-year-old girl, weighed 76 lb at the start of treatment, down 25 lb from her usual weight. The other, a seventeen-year-old, weighed 69 lb, which was 22 lb below what she usually weighed. The therapeutic strategy called for ignoring all comments the girls would make related to such physical complaints as headaches, nausea, or cramps. This extinction procedure resulted in a drastic reduction of these complaints, but it did not increase food intake or body weight, suggesting that food refusal was not maintained by contingent attention from the environment. Only when verbal praise for food intake and such pleasurable activities as watching TV or taking walks were made contingent on food intake and weight gain, did the girls' body weights increase to near their normal levels. Before this reinforcement regimen had been introduced, the girls had spent time in a hospital setting where they were exposed to personal attention, persuasion, and attempts to reduce their fear of obesity. Since this had not resulted in weight gain, Leitenberg et al. (1968) conclude that contingent reinforcement was responsible for the improvement, and they state that food refusal appears to be an avoidance behavior and not a response pattern that is maintained by positive reinforcement. The latter assertion is based on the observation that food refusal failed to abate when it was being ignored during the period when physical complaints were undergoing extinction.

When the eating behavior of an adolescent with normal intelligence is to be brought under control, explicitly spelled out contingencies ("if you gain weight, you can watch TV") which are consistently enforced appear capable of reducing food refusal. When weight loss is a result not of noneating but of vomiting and when the individual is not a bright but a severely retarded adolescent or an infant, treatment must take a different form. Kohlenberg (1970) and Luckey, Watson, and Musick (1968)—working with severely retarded children—and Lang and Melamed (1969)—who treated an infant—approached chronic ruminative vomiting through an avoidance-conditioning paradigm. The somewhat drastic technique of introducing punishment contingent on vomiting is called for when, as in these cases, the continuing loss of body weight represents a threat to the child's life. Kohlenberg (1970) succeeded in reducing vomiting in a nonverbal mongoloid by delivering a shock to the thigh contingent on stomach tension which had been observed to precede the actual vomiting. This approach was later supplemented by confining the subject to a chair contingent on having vomited and resulted in a weight gain of $10\frac{1}{2}$ lb in 25 days. As is frequently the case when punishment of an undesired response is used in the absence of positive reinforcement of its functionally reciprocal desired response, vomiting again became a problem about a year later, highlighting the fact that while punishment is an effective emergency measure, it does not constitute treatment in the absence of a more positive approach.

In the case of a normally developing young child, as opposed to a retardate, the positive consequences normally contingent on non-vomiting behavior appear to support such behavior once the vomiting has been suppressed by avoidance conditioning. Lang and Melamed (1969) report on a nine-month-old male infant whose ruminative vomiting had reduced his weight to 12 lb (from 17 lb at six months of age). This infant had developed normally until his fifth month when he first began vomiting. The problem increased in severity to the point where the child vomited within 10 to 15 minutes after every meal. The onset of the problem coincided with the mother's indisposition because of a broken ankle which had forced the family to live for several weeks in the home of the maternal grandparents. There is a report of friction between the mother and her own adoptive mother regarding the care of the child, but no details as to possible conditions under which the vomiting might have been learned are included in the child's history. The vomiting resulted in three brief hospitalizations for the purpose of various tests, including exploratory surgery; but none of these revealed a medical reason for the problem, nor did any of several treatment approaches reduce the frequency of vomiting. Conditioning procedures were introduced as a last resort and because the infant's life was endangered.

Treatment consisted of delivery of an electric shock through an electrode attached to the child's calf as soon as electromyographic recording indicated that vomiting was about to occur. The shock was paired with a loud tone, and the effect of the treatment was dramatic. After two sessions shock was rarely required, and by the sixth session the infant was no longer vomiting. He began to gain weight during the treatment and continued to improve thereafter. One month after discharge from the hospital he weighed 21 lb, and 5 months later his weight was 26 lb, 1 oz. He was eating well and not vomiting, and a physician described him as alert, active, and attentive. He continued to thrive when followed up 1 year after treatment. Coincident with the successful conditioning therapy, the child's positive social behavior had increased; he had become more responsive to adults, smiled more frequently, and seemed to be more interested in toys and games than he had been previously. There seemed to have been no adverse consequences to the avoidance conditioning, and positive reinforcers normally available in the social environment appear to have been sufficient to maintain normal, nonruminative behavior.

MASTURBATION IN PUBLIC

Masturbation, like eating, is a behavior that carries its own, inherent, and positive consequences; but unlike eating, it is not prone to be encouraged, rewarded, or modeled by a parent. Yet for both eating and masturbation appropriate self-control is the goal and usual outcome of socialization. It is the lack of such control which leads these problems to be classified as behavior deficits. In the course of socialization the child must learn that genital self-stimulation is inappropriate when practiced in public. In this sense, the social proscription is the same as that imposed on nosepicking, and it is a reflection on the values of our society that children do not get referred for professional help because they pick their noses in public. It is, of course, easier to teach a child not to pick his nose than not to masturbate because nosepicking does not carry powerful, inherent positive reinforcement.

When masturbation takes place only in nonpublic situations, that is, when it is under the stimulus control of these situations (such as the child's bedroom), the behavior is not a problem, and only an intrusive parent would be aware of it. If a child spends "too much" time closeted in a room so that a parent would suspect that he is engaging in excessive masturbation, one must inquire why other activities and interpersonal contacts are aversive or less reinforcing than the positive consequences of masturbation. Once the balance of reinforcements is shifted so that the child can have gratification in the presence of stimuli that control suppression of masturbation, the problem should disappear. At the same time it is obvious that a child who has had limited interpersonal contacts while he was engaged in his solitary activity will need to learn peer-relationship skills before such relationship can become gratifying.

As a reflection of the fact that masturbation is a taboo topic in our society, there is no systematic, controlled research on genital self-stimulation in children and, in fact, relatively little mention of it in the clinical literature.

ENURESIS AND ENCOPRESIS

Lack of appropriate control over the elimination of urine (*enuresis*) and feces (*encopresis*) has received considerable attention in the psychological literature, at least in part because Freudian tradition held that the conditions under which this control is learned ("toilet training") play a critical role in personality development. When a mother is faced with the task of teaching her child to eliminate in a place and under conditions his society happens to consider "appropriate," she uses the same skills (or lack of skill) at teaching that she brings to other aspects of child rearing. As such, she has an impact not only on the child's specific behaviors with regard to toilet functions but also on all the other behaviors, the constellation of which we come to call "personality." An impatient mother who insists on early and quick bowel control and punishes noncompliance is also likely to insist on and model such behavioral qualities as neatness, cleanliness, frugality, and orderliness. When her child later exhibits these qualities, he does so not necessarily because of the way he was toilet trained but because of the similar manner in which the mother who toilet trained him also taught him other behaviors.

As is true of so many other psychological disorders, there is a problem in defining difficulties with elimination. It is, again, a rather arbitrary decision whether or not to call occasional bed-wetting by a five-year-old a psychological problem. What is "occasional"? And at what age does it cease to be normal and become a problem? Among the school-age children studied by Lapouse and Monk (1959), 8 percent wet their beds at least once a month; yet these were normal children, if not being a patient at a psychiatric clinic can be taken as a definition of normality. There are families in parts of the United States where bed-wetting at any age is accepted as an expected, unremarkable event, and there are others who become concerned when a child of three is unable to sleep without wetting. In the final analysis, it is the child's environment which defines the problem; once any behavior is classified in the rubric of "problem," the responses of the environment make it a problem behavior, no matter what cutoff point or definition textbook writers might offer.

Enuresis and the related but rarer disorder, encopresis, are encountered in two forms—chronic and regressive. In both forms, wetting usually occurs at night (nocturnal enuresis or bed-wetting), but in more serious cases the child may also wet during the day. Encopresis, or soiling, on the other hand, usually occurs during the day and is often associated with periods of excessive bowel retention.

In *chronic enuresis* the child has never learned to hold his urine and to micturate only in appropriate places. In *regressive enuresis* the child will have learned urinary control at one time but has resumed wetting some time later. Such regression can be conceptualized in terms of a response hierarchy in which response patterns of increasing maturity have been acquired sequentially. At the top of the hierarchy the prepotent and most likely, but most recently learned, response to a distended bladder is to inhibit the innate elimination response until the appropriate stimulus conditions of the toilet are present. Like other instrumental responses, the sequence hold-wait-seek toilet-urinate was probably learned and maintained by positive consequences. During acquisition in childhood, these consequences may have included maternal attention and praise for being mature and self-sufficient. If these consequences should then be withdrawn before the mature response is fully established and maintained by the negative reinforcement of tension release and by positive consequences such as pride in achievement which the child can deliver to himself, one would predict the mature response pattern to undergo extinction, with a less mature pattern—lower on the hierarchy—(i.e., wetting) becoming prepotent.

When a child resumes wetting after an earlier period of having been toilet-trained, the consequences of the regressive response tend to be maternal consternation which, despite its negative content, is a form of attention and hence a potential reinforcer for the wetting behavior. Some mothers may attempt to punish the child for wetting, but since such punishment is administered a considerable time after the wetting response was made (i.e., when the wet bed is discovered in the morning), it is bound to be ineffective. Negative attention or punishment or both are unlikely to reestablish the desired "dry night" behavior at the prepotent position in the hierarchy. On the contrary, the attention may, in fact, strengthen the wetting behavior.

In order to teach the two responses that together represent adaptive toileting behavior—"hold" and "release in right place"—these responses must be strengthened by positive reinforcement, while their inappropriate reciprocals are weakened through non-reinforcement (extinction) or negative consequences (punishment). It is only in this combination and when administered as soon after the response as possible that punishment can have the desired effect. Even when properly timed, punishment alone is effective only in the inhibiting ("hold") aspect of the response sequence; it cannot develop the desired behavior of going to the toilet and eliminating. Since inhibition alone will ultimately be overwhelmed by the increasing physiological bladder tension with resulting elimination, punishment, when used, must be paired with teaching the positive response.

In encopresis, as was pointed out, one frequently finds periods of excessive fecal retention alternating with periods of soiling. It may be that these are children who have learned only the "hold" part of the response sequence, possibly because their toilet training emphasized aversive control (punishment). Extended periods of bowel retention can result in a hardening of fecal matter because of moisture absorption so that the stools become so impacted that defecation becomes painful. To avoid this pain, the child may continue his retention until, in some instances, defecation becomes physically impossible and medical intervention is required in order to induce evacuation.

Aversive control can, under certain circumstances, bring about the suppression of a response, but the more likely responses learned under these conditions are avoidance and escape. Some encopretic children learn to hide the evidence of their soiling, secreting dirty underwear in the most ingenious places—much to the understandable distress of their family. When a positive response is to be established, in this case associating the internal cues of bladder or bowel tension with going to the toilet to eliminate, this positive response must be explicitly taught. When the contingencies are wrong, the wrong behavior will be strengthened. This was demonstrated in a case reported by Lal and Lindsley (1968). A three-year-old boy had developed chronic constipation. Observation revealed that whenever the boy failed to eliminate, his parents would shower him with affection on the mistaken assumption that his constipation was the result of his feeling insecure and needing more love. With receiving affection thus contingent on *not* eliminating, the boy's condition became worse. Improvement came quickly once the parents were instructed to place the boy on the toilet and to leave him alone until he called to indicate that he had defecated and *then* to praise and caress him and to permit him to engage in the highly desired privilege of playing with his water toys in the bathtub.

The discussion thus far may have led to the impression that the only trouble with an enuretic or encopretic child is that he eliminates too often in inappropriate places and that he merely has to learn the hold-wait-eliminate in toilet sequence of responses in order to be rid of his problem. By the time a child who does not display age-appropriate toilet behavior comes to clinical attention, he is likely to have acquired at least some conditioned anxiety to stimuli associated with wetting or soiling. Some of these stimuli, such as the sensation associated with sphincter release and urine passing through the urethra, are the same whether the elimination takes place in an appropriate or inappropriate place. Anxiety which has become associated with these stimuli thus represents an incompatible response when it is elicited while the child is on the toilet. One aspect of treating enuresis is thus the discrimination learning whereby toilet cues will no longer elicit the anxiety response and its toilet-avoiding consequences.

Another concomitant of wetting and soiling is found in the perceptions the child forms of himself and of his capacity to cope with problems. Having failed to learn what "any baby can learn," that is, to control his bladder or bowels, a child is likely to see himself as inadequate, incompetent, or worthless. Since his condition is also likely to limit his interactions with peers (no sleeping at a friend's house, no overnight camp), this area of his life also tends to be disrupted. These conditions are reversed once the child's enuresis is successfully treated, and there tends to be a marked improvement in areas such as peer relations, school behavior, and general adjustment even when none of these are subject to direct treatment (Baker, 1969).

Compton (1968) addressed a study to the spontaneous changes accompanying conditioning treatment of enuretics. He obtained a measure of self-concept from 40 enuretics and 40 controls between the ages of eight and eighteen both before and after the enuretics received treatment. Before treatment the self-concept scores of the enuretics were significantly below those of the controls, but for the 33 successfully treated cases these scores improved to the point where they were the same as those of the controls. While it is tempting to use studies of this nature as support for the contention that such personality characteristics of children with psychophysiological disorders as shyness, immaturity, dependency, or anxiety are not the causes but the effects of asthma, obesity, or enuresis, research by Baker (1969) or Compton (1968) says nothing about the direction of causality in the development of these disorders. These studies do, however, throw doubt on the opposite contention that these psychophysiological problems are so intimately tied to personality states that they can only be treated by methods that focus on the modification of personality.

RECAPITULATION

The biological functions of the body, the physiological conditions, play a role in every form of human behavior, in every behavior disorder. In some behavior disorders the role of physiological functions is more prominent than in others, and such disorders can be singled out and called *psychophysiological disorders.* Asthma is a classic example of such a disorder, and there have been many speculations about the interaction and direction of causality between environmental and biological factors. Research suggests that in some children asthmatic attacks are under the control of environmental stimuli, but little is known about what it is that makes these children susceptible to these effects. Overeating and food refusal are often related to external stimuli, particularly parental behavior, and this seems also the case where a child lacks appropriate control over eliminatory processes as in enuresis and encopresis. In these disorders it is useful to differentiate between chronic and regressive cases; for in the former, the child has never learned appropriate control, while in the latter these controls, once learned, have become lost.

With psychophysiological disorders, and particularly with asthma, it is difficult to decide whether one is dealing with deficient or with excess behavior, and so it seems appropriate that this discussion stands at that point in this book where we turn our consideration from the former to the latter.

PART III

EXCESS BEHAVIOR

9

AGGRESSIVE
BEHAVIOR

In the socialization of the child no response pattern has more important implications, both from the point of view of the child's own adaptation and of its effect on society, than that involving aggression. The vicissitudes of helping a child learn to behave appropriately in this realm are evidenced by the fact that children with maladaptive behavior patterns involving aggressive responses make up a large proportion of any clinic population (Gilbert, 1957). In order to understand this problem so as to be able to deal with it from a therapeutic and preventative point of view, it is necessary to arrive at a meaningful formulation of this complex issue.

AGGRESSION IS A RESPONSE

Aggression is best viewed as an overt response, a response, as Buss (1961) defined it, that delivers a noxious stimulus to another person. The noxious quality of the stimulus can take a variety of forms; hence aggression takes a variety of forms. It can involve the inflicting of physical pain, the withholding of reinforcement, the damaging of property, the presentation of irritating stimuli, the blocking of a consummatory response, or the presentation of negative evaluations.

This listing, which is by no means exhaustive, immediately suggests the relative nature of this definition. Pain inflicted in the course of medical treatment, reinforcement withheld as part of a teaching program, and the parent's interruption of a toddler's consummatory response of swallowing a marble are not considered instances of aggression. Similarly, what is an irritating auditory stimulus to one listener is music to another, and a negative evaluation can be a term endearment under certain circumstances.

Such relativity indicates that under certain conditions a given response is labeled *aggression,* while, under different conditions, the same response carries a different label. One is thus led to the recognition that aggression is not an absolute entity but a relative concept whose use is a function of social convention : A response is labeled as aggressive if agents of the social-labeling process consider it capable of inflicting pain, damage, or loss to another individual *and* if the circumstances are judged not to warrant such an outcome. As Bandura and Walters (1963), who first proposed this definition, point out, this labeling process involves not only a social value judgment regarding the outcome but also the identification of a response sequence as possessing characteristics that are likely to inflict pain, damage, or loss on others. One of these characteristics, but by no means the only one, is the high magnitude or intensity of the response (Walters & Brown, 1964).

Numerous examples can be given in which a specific response (e.g., pat-on-the-cheek) is labeled as *affectionate* when it is emitted at low intensity, but called *aggressive* (slap-in-the-face) when a topographically similar response, that is, one with manifestly similar characteristics, is emitted with higher intensity. Clearly, as Walters (1964) took pains to stress, not every high-magnitude response will be labeled as aggressive, but a child who emits high-magnitude responses at a high frequency is more likely to be viewed as behaving in an aggressive manner than the child whose frequency of such responses is lower. This "high magnitude" formulation of aggression and the research that has been generated by it will be examined in some detail after several other implications have been considered.

Intensity of response is one of the temperamental characteristics which were discussed in Chapter 3 in dealing with behavioral style. Observable from birth on, and probably innate, general intensity of response may contribute to the development of children with response tendencies likely to be labeled as aggressive. This is not to say that aggressive behavior is congenital or hereditary; it merely means that a child who has a characteristically high intensity of responding has a greater likelihood of being called *aggressive* than his peer who emits responses at lower intensities. At least of equal importance with behavioral style in the development of a child who emits aggressive responses is the value system of his social environment which not only labels his behavior selectively but also introduces contingencies that will strengthen or weaken the responses that it classifies as aggressive.

With aggression viewed as an overt response it is necessary to differentiate it from a motivational factor that is often correlated with aggression but is neither synonymous with nor invariably accompanying aggression. This motivational (emotional) factor is a physiological arousal state generally called *anger* or *rage*. This arousal state appears to be elicited by certain stimuli, particularly those involving attack (aggression directed against the individual) and frustration (blocking of a response sequence before the consummatory response is reached). It is not clear whether anger is physiologically different from fear (Buss, 1961); therefore it is more parsimonious to view it as an arousal state to which the label *anger* has been applied. As a correlate of an aggression response, anger can strengthen this response when the arousal is reduced after the aggression response has been emitted.

Aggression can thus be strengthened in line with the negative reinforcement paradigm in that a noxious tension state is terminated contingent on the response being emitted. The other mode of strengthening aggression is through positive reinforcement when the individual encounters a positive consequence (gets something he wants) contingent on emitting an aggressive response. It is not at all unlikely that the apparent universality of aggression and the obdurate nature of the response in the face of attempts to modify it are a function of the ready availability of eliciting stimuli and reinforcing conditions.

THE LEARNING OF AGGRESSION

Once aggression is defined as a response, it becomes possible to study the conditions under which this response is learned, and when the conditions are known, it should be possible to modify and ultimately control this socially disruptive behavior. It can be shown that aggression, like any other response, is strengthened by reinforcement and that it undergoes extinction when reinforcement is withdrawn (Cowan & Walters, 1963). Both stimulus and response generalization have been demonstrated (Walters & Brown, 1963; Lovaas, 1961a), and discrimination-learning has been shown to be effective (Bandura & Walters, 1963). As with other instrumental responses, modeling serves as an important source of learning, and this may well be an explanation for the apparent paradox that parents who use physical punishment (aggression) in their attempt to control the aggressive behavior of their children tend to raise highly aggressive children (Bandura & Walters, 1959). Punishment usually occurs with some delay, and thus at an inefficient point in time, and the parent who attacks his child models aggressive behavior under emotion-related stimulus conditions and so the child may well learn to make aggression responses under these conditions. Since the influence of models appears particularly great when the observer is emotionally aroused (Schachter & Singer, 1962), the punishing situation may be especially potent for the learning of aggression.

The High-Magnitude Theory

The high-magnitude theory of aggression proposed by Bandura and Walters (1963) holds that the cultural definition of aggression is in part a function of the intensity with which the response is emitted and that response intensity can be increased by delayed reinforcement (frustration). The theory also maintains that a given high-magnitude response may be learned under conditions where it is not judged to be aggressive but that when the same response is emitted under different circumstances, it can be regarded as an instance of aggression.

The above assertion was put to experimental test in a study conducted by Walters and Brown (1964), who trained boys from kindergarten, first, and second grades to emit either high-magnitude or low-magnitude responses in doll-punching or lever-pressing tasks on which they were differentially reinforced. Following each training session every subject was paired with another boy of the same age, and the two were invited to engage in competitive games requiring a good deal of body contact. The behavior of the experimental child in each pair was observed and scored for such responses as butting, kneeing, elbowing, kicking, punching, pulling, pushing, etc. The results were clearly in line with the hypothesis, for the children trained under high-intensity conditions emitted significantly more aggression responses during testing than did those who had been trained under low-intensity conditions. It will be recalled that the responses used during the training sessions were hitting and lever-pressing, while the behaviors scored as "aggression" in the testing sessions did not include hitting and certainly not lever-pressing. The generalization from training to testing involved not only the nature of the response but also the characteristic of intensity.

While the games used by Walters and Brown in the testing procedure were highly competitive, they did not entail frustration in the sense of either delayed reinforcement or interrupted goal-directed behavior. The pretraining alone seemed sufficient to bring about differential degrees of aggression depending on whether a particular child had been given high-intensity or low-intensity training preceding his participation in the games. A study by Davitz (1952) had used two of these very games for aggression training, suggesting the demand characteristics of these games; yet even in the face of these characteristics the children with low-intensity training emitted significantly fewer aggressive responses while engaged in these games.

The Davitz games are "cover that spot," "scalp," and "break the ball." Their respective goals are to cover a small "x" on the floor with some part of one's body when the game is terminated, to tear a piece of cloth tied around the arms of the competitors from the opponent's arm while protecting one's own "scalp," and to break the other player's ping pong balls while protecting one's own ball. Using these games Davitz (1952) trained 20 boys and girls between the ages of seven and nine to be aggressive, while a comparison group received "constructive training" involving the drawing of murals and the completion of jigsaw puzzles. Prior to the seven 30-minute training sessions, the children had been observed during 18 minutes of free play which were recorded on motion picture film. A similar period of free play followed a "frustration session." In this the children were led to believe that they would be shown a series of five films. After the first reel had been shown, each subject was given a bar of candy, but the second reel was interrupted at a climactic point and the candy was taken away. During the filmed free-play session following this frustration situation the children who had been trained to behave aggressively in the competitive games behaved significantly more aggressively than did those trained in constructive activities. What is more, the subjects who had been trained to engage in constructive behavior behaved more constructively after the frustration than did the subjects who had been trained for aggression. This study strongly suggests that frustration does not automatically lead to aggression but that the stimuli involved in a frustration situation tend to elicit whatever response pattern happens to be dominant in a given subject's response hierarchy. Since the children in the Davitz experiment were exposed to the frustration and then tested in the same small group of 4 with whom they had been previously in their training sessions, it can be assumed that they provided the stimulus complex for each other that controlled the response pattern elicited by the frustration situation. Inasmuch as constructive play is by and large incompatible with aggressive behavior, constructive activity may well serve as the response pattern which, when sufficiently strengthened, can take the place of aggressive behavior provided aggression is simultaneously weakened by nonreinforcement.

Punishment and Aggression

As was pointed out earlier, physical punishment for aggression can have the paradoxical consequence of increasing aggression because the parent who delivers the punishment serves as a model for aggression under highly emotional circumstances. A study by Hollenberg and Sperry (1951) bears on this and related issues. These investigators studied the behavior of 53 children between the ages of three and six years in four 15-minute doll-play sessions, using a doll house and standard doll family. The play behavior was observed and scored for frequency and intensity. On the basis of interviews with the children's mothers, two measures of home experiences were obtained. These dealt with frustration and punishment for aggression.

When 15 of the children whose mothers had been rated as high in punishment were compared with an equal number of children from low-punishment homes, it was found that the children who were highly punished for aggression at home emitted aggressive behaviors during doll play more frequently and more intensely than children who had experienced milder punishment at home. An analysis of the interrelationship between punishment and frustration revealed that children from a high-punishment–high-frustration background tended to emit more aggression responses during doll-play sessions than did the children from a low-punishment–low-frustration background. Hollenberg and Sperry interpreted their findings in the context of drive-reduction theory and the conflict model, but their data can be as readily seen as supporting the modeling paradigm of Bandura and Walters (1963).

Another aspect of the Hollenberg and Sperry research dealt with the effects of punishment in the doll play situation itself. For this purpose, 12 children were assigned to the *experimentally punished* group and 11 children to the *control* group. All of the children participated in the four permissive doll-play sessions, but the experimentally punished group received verbal disapproval for each aggressive response during the second of the four sessions. In the presence of the permissive adult both frequency and intensity of aggression on the part of the children in the control group increased over the four sessions. For the children in the experimentally punished group however, there was no increase in aggression from Session I to Session II and a marked decrease during Session III. The negative social consequence (verbal reprimand) had only a short-range effect on the aggression responses, for, by the time of Session IV, the frequency of aggression responses emitted by the punished children approached the frequency for the control group.

While only three of the differences recorded by Hollenberg and Sperry reached statistical significance and even though the interview-based ratings of home frustration and punishment are of limited reliability, their work suggests that aggressive responses are strengthened when they occur in the presence of a permissive adult. They are weakened when followed by *verbal* indications of disapproval but strengthened, particularly for emission in situations away from home, when aggressive behaviors are followed by severe *physical* punishment in the home. It would thus seem that the parent who does not model aggression but consistently indicates his disapproval of aggression will raise a child who will emit a low rate of aggression responses both at home and away from the home. Beyond this it would follow from available research on learning that the strengthening of aggression-incompatible responses and the teaching of constructive alternative responses to stimulus situations which have come to control aggression should lead to a low incidence of aggressive behavior.

Conditions Favoring Aggression

Frustration is a stimulus configuration which often controls aggressive responses. In fact, in our culture it is so often observed that frustration precedes aggression that for several decades the frustration-aggression hypothesis of the Yale group (Dollard et al., 1939), who held that aggression is always the consequence of frustration, was viewed as defining the necessary and sufficient conditions for aggression. Note that this formulation does not state that frustration is *always* followed by aggression, but the frustration-aggression hypothesis was often interpreted as if it proposed this causal sequence.

The word *frustration,* as used in everyday language, carries connotations of a state in an individual who has been thwarted in some action—one says "I feel frustrated." From a behavioral point of view it is best to limit the use of "frustration" to designating a stimulus configuration represented by external events surrounding the blocking of a response sequence. When frustration is used in this way, aggression can be viewed as one of many responses that an individual might learn to emit when this stimulus configuration is present. Conversely, the response labeled as aggression can be learned to a great variety of external stimuli, such as the command "fight!" or the sound of a gong in a boxing ring.

The blocking of a response sequence before the goal is reached ("frustration," for short) has two characteristics that raise the probability that it will come to control responses that are likely to be labeled as aggressive. One characteristic is that the blocked goal can often be reached, the frustration removed, when a high-intensity response, such as pushing, is emitted. The other characteristic is that response blocking tends to elicit an arousal state which increases the probability that any response emitted under these circumstances will have relatively high intensity. If, in the child's reinforcement history, such high-intensity responses (pushing, hitting, kicking, etc.) are repeatedly followed by attaining the blocked goal or other reinforcement, such responses are strengthened and likely to be emitted whenever the child encounters a similar stimulus configuration ("frustration"). Inasmuch as our culture defines high-intensity pushing, hitting, and kicking as "aggression," the frustration-aggression sequence can be observed with great frequency. This does not mean, however, that aggression is the innate or inevitable consequence of frustration. It can, in fact, be demonstrated (e.g., Block and Martin, 1955) that some children consistently respond to frustration in a manner our culture defines as "constructive," and it would seem to follow from the work of Davitz (1952) that careful discrimination teaching can develop a child who behaves in a prosocial fashion whenever he encounters frustration.

We know that some learning is facilitated when the learner is in a state of emotional arousal (Palermo et al., 1956). This not only enhances the likelihood of the acquisition of the frustration-aggression sequence but it also has bearing on the aggressive behavior of disturbed children who may be seen as more frequently aroused or more highly aroused, or both, than those in the general population. A study by Cowan and Walters (1963) bears on this issue. They compared thirty boys, residents in an institution for "emotionally disturbed children" and ranging in age from eight to thirteen years, with an equal number of noninstitutionalized controls from public school. The subjects were reinforced with colored glass marbles for emitting hitting responses aimed at the stomach of an automated Bobo clown. One group received reinforcement on a continuous schedule, another on a 1 to 3 fixed-ratio schedule, and a third group was on a 1 to 6 fixed-ratio schedule. After a subject had made eighteen responses, reinforcement was discontinued and he was allowed to continue responding until he desired to stop. During this extinction period, the institutionalized children gave significantly more responses and continued to respond for a longer time than the noninstitutionalized children.

Under two of the three reinforcement conditions the institutionalized children responded more rapidly than the noninstitutionalized children. During both acquisition and extinction the institutionalized children performed in a manner that suggests a greater effectiveness of reinforcement procedures for this group. Cowan and Walters point out that the institutionalized subjects became highly excited when placed in the experimental situation and that this excitement frequently lasted throughout the experimental sessions. The authors suggest that the greater effectiveness of reinforcers under conditions of arousal is due to the fact that arousal restricts attention and thus places a subject's behavior more under control of salient environmental cues.

While this formulation is consonant with other studies, particularly those from the area of vicarious learning (Bandura & Rosenthal, 1966), there is an alternate explanation to the Cowan and Walters findings than one that focuses on the effectiveness of reinforcers that were dispensed during the training trials. The institutionalized subjects were described as having been referred to the hospital because they presented behavior problems to the community. These behavior problems presumably included a high proportion of aggressive behaviors so that, in other words, aggressive responses have a high probability of occurrence in the repertoire of these institutionalized children. Such responses, as Premack (1959) has suggested, are reinforcing in their own right so that the institutionalized subjects may well have received two reinforcers: the hitting response *and* the glass marble. This would account for both the higher response rate and the resistance to extinction without invoking the hypothesis about arousal level. To test the latter it would be necessary to teach disturbed children a response that is not likely to be high in their hierarchy. It would also be necessary to control for the differential consequences to stopping the clown-hitting response (extinction) inasmuch as institutionalized children are then taken back to the ward while the school child is returned to his classroom. If returning to the ward is a negative consequence, sustained activity on the experimental apparatus in the absence of reinforcement might be avoidance behavior and not resistance to extinction.

The reinforcing capacity of hitting responses aimed at a plastic clown is highlighted in a paper by Hops and Walters (1963) who point out that during the operant phase of their study, that is, before reinforcement was introduced, many children reached a level of response that may have been near their physiological limit. This study also suggests that the rate of hitting responses in a Bobo clown situation is an aspect of the child's general activity level. Earlier in this chapter we pointed out that a child who has a characteristically high activity level has a greater likelihood of being called *aggressive.* The Hops and Walters results may bear on this point. They show that there is a wide range of individual differences among children's activity level and that there are high correlations between response rates under different reinforcement conditions that reflect considerable intraindividual consistency. Children who have a high activity level emit a high rate of responses under many different conditions, and when response possibilities are restricted, as in an experimental Bobo clown situation, these children emit a high rate of hitting responses. It would be fallacious to conclude from observing the behavior of such children that they are "aggressive." Before one can draw conclusions about a child's generalized aggressive response tendency, one would have to demonstrate that he emits a higher rate of aggressive responses than of other responses that are equally possible in a given situation.

An experiment in which the child subjects were able to choose between an aggressive and a nonaggressive response was conducted by Lovaas (1961a). The aggressive response was defined as a bar press that activated a doll apparatus so that one boy doll would hit another boy doll on the head with a stick. The nonaggressive response involved a bar press that activated a ball game apparatus in such a way that a ball would be thrown to the top of a cage from where it would return through obstacles to its original position. The experimental manipulation took the form of showing the subjects two films—one was depicting human-like cartoon figures in highly aggressive interaction, while the other was a peaceful scene showing a bear family in humanlike play. The children who had been shown the aggressive film engaged in significantly more play behavior with the hitting dolls than did those children who had been shown the nonaggressive film. The results thus give evidence for an increase in aggressive responses as a function of exposure to film-mediated aggression, suggesting that the viewing of aggressive films is likely to make children more aggressive.

The relationship between aggressive behavior in real life situations and activity with a mechanical toy that symbolizes human aggression was demonstrated by Parton (1964). He used a boxing doll device which was activated by the squeezing of a trigger so that the doll that was manipulated by the subject could be made to hit the opponent doll. The apparatus was so constructed that the experimenter could cause the opponent doll to hit the subject's doll in return and it further permitted him to control either doll's falling down. Parton demonstrated an interaction between the children's behavior with the boxing doll device and their history of peer aggression, as measured on a peer-rating measure of aggression developed by Walder et al. (1961). The children with high peer-aggression scores held their doll in the fighting range under the condition in which the opponent doll was hitting for more time than any other group under any other condition. On the other hand, the subjects with low peer-aggression scores held their doll in the fight range for less time under conditions when the opponent doll was hitting than under the condition when the opponent doll was not hitting. The overall result of this study also reveals the highest hitting rate under conditions where the opponent doll would hit back, and the lowest rate under the condition where the only consequence of hitting was to see the opponent doll knocked down. This would suggest that counteraggression is a stronger reinforcer for an aggressive response than mere "victory." This, however, is not compatible with the observations of nursery school behavior reported by Patterson, Littman, and Bricker (1967) who found a decrease in aggressive behavior when the victim retaliated. The heightened performance under conditions of retaliation found in the Parton study may thus be an artifact of the doll-play situation in that a trigger-squeeze response is probably more strongly reinforced by the consequence of seeing two dolls hit one another than by the consequence of having one doll knock down the other.

While doll-play aggression is no more than an analogue of interpersonal aggression, a second study by Lovaas (1961b), using the apparatus previously described, lends further support to the utility of doll play as a device for studying aggression responses. This study demonstrated the generalization of aggressive responses from the verbal to the nonverbal mode. Two groups of children were differentially reinforced for making aggressive or nonaggressive verbal responses in the presence of a "bad" and a "good" doll. Seven subjects were reinforced with trinkets for emitting such responses as "bad doll" and "dirty doll," while the other seven subjects were similarly reinforced for emitting nonaggressive verbal statements. When these children were then given the choice of playing with the aforementioned hitting-dolls or bouncing-ball equipment, those who had been reinforced for verbal aggression showed a significant preference for playing with the hitting-dolls apparatus.

"Catharsis" and Aggression

Taken together, the two studies by Lovaas (1961a, 1961b) would seem to argue strongly against the validity of the catharsis hypothesis which holds that a child can "get aggressive impulses out of his system" by either giving these presumed impulses verbal expression or by the vicarious experience of observing aggression depicted in the form of a film or television program. Children who had been reinforced for aggressive verbal statements made more, rather than fewer, aggressive motor responses, compared to their base-rate performance, and the same was true of children who had watched an aggressive film.

Three related studies, conducted by Mallick and McCandless (1966), were specifically designed to test the hypothesis that aggressive play has no cathartic effect. The three studies were similar in design. A total of 168 children in the third grade were asked to engage in a moderately simple block-construction task. They were told that they could earn 5 cents for each of five tasks, provided each was completed within a time limit. A child of the same sex as the subject, attending the sixth grade, served as the experimenters' confederate and had the task of interfering with the subject's activities in such a way that the subject was frustrated in completing his tasks on time. Sarcastic remarks were interspersed with this interference. In the nonfrustration condition, the confederate helped the subjects complete their tasks, but no monetary reward was either promised or given.

Following the block-construction task, which lasted for 5 minutes, all subjects entered one of three interpolated tasks which lasted for 8 minutes. Depending on the condition to which a particular subject had been assigned, the interpolated task consisted of shooting at a target on which a picture of a child of the same age and sex as the confederate had been placed, engaging in social talk with the experimenter, or being given a "reasonable interpretation of the frustrator's behavior." This interpretation consisted of indicating to the subject "that the frustrator was sleepy, upset, and would probably have been more cooperative if the subject had offered him two of the five nickles." The third phase of the study consisted of a behavioral measure of aggression. All subjects were given the opportunity to "punish" the confederate, either by pushing a button that presumably administered a mild shock to him or by pushing one of two buttons that would either help or hinder the confederate in a task he was presumably attempting to complete. The "shock" situation prevailed in one of the three studies, while the other measure was used in the remaining two. For the second and third study, Mallick and McCandless also administered a "like-dislike" scale on which the subject was asked to indicate his attitude toward the confederate. This scale was administered both before and after the interpolated 8-minute task.

Analysis of the like-dislike ratings revealed that the frustration treatment (interference with assigned task) had a highly significant effect in that the children in the frustration groups disliked the experimenters' confederate much more than did those in the nonfrustration groups. For those whose interpolated phase entailed either social talk or aggressive play, the dislike rating was not reduced, while those who had received the "interpretation" showed a significant change in the direction of more positive attitudes. The behavioral measures of aggression (pushing the "shocking" or "hindering" button) showed that frustrated subjects had significantly higher mean aggression scores than comparable treatment groups of nonfrustrated subjects. Again, as on the attitude scale, the group that had been given the "interpretation" showed significantly fewer aggression responses than the subjects in the other two frustration groups; in fact, they did not differ in their responses from the subjects in the nonfrustration groups.

The catharsis hypothesis would predict that a child made angry by the frustration situation and given a chance to express aggression in the target-shooting session would show less residual aggression on a subsequent measure than a child who had no opportunity at "catharsis." Contrary to this prediction, the interpolated aggressive play did not reduce aggression as measured by the button pressing. In fact, for those subjects who had not been frustrated, aggressive play actually increased subsequent aggression toward the non-frustrating playmate.

The findings thus suggest that aggressive play not only fails to have a "cathartic" effect but that, as reinforcement theory would predict, aggressive play in the presence of a permissive adult actually leads to increased aggression and that the verbal expression of hostility, as facilitated by the like-dislike ratings, also increases subsequent behavioral aggression.

Mallick and McCandless view the results from their interpretation condition as showing the cathartic, aggression-reducing effect of a "reasonable interpretation." The reduction of aggression on both the attitude and the behavioral measures is difficult to conceive as "catharsis" in the traditional pressure-releasing sense of the hydraulic analogy. The subjects under this condition could not express or act out their anger; instead they listened to some explanatory statements from the experimenter. Since the statements entailed apologies for the confederate's behavior, coupled with placing blame on the subject for not having offered the confederate a portion of his potential monetary gain, they may well have carried the implication "don't be angry at him, it's really your fault." Rather than having cathartic value, this message was more likely to indicate the adult experimenters' nonpermissive, potentially punitive attitude toward expressing aggression against the confederate. Inasmuch as the experimenter's permissive presence during the aggressive play seemed to have increased subsequent aggression, it would seem reasonable to assume that the nonpermissive attitude implied in the so-called interpretation served to increase suppression of aggressive responses, a development which can hardly be viewed as "catharsis." This conclusion is all the more plausible because the subjects in this study are described as coming principally from the middle and upper class; that is, they were the children for whom the kind of statements made by the experimenter about the confederate's behavior probably represent well-established discriminative stimuli for suppressing aggressive responses.

AGGRESSION AS AN ASSERTIVE BEHAVIOR

The high-magnitude theory of aggression proposed by Bandura and Walters (1963) states that any response that is emitted at high magnitude or intensity is likely to be labeled as aggressive if it has the potential to inflict pain, damage, or loss to another person under circumstances not warranting such an outcome. It will be noted that this formulation does not make emotional arousal a necessary condition for the definition of aggression.

A somewhat different approach to defining aggression is taken by Patterson, Littman, and Bricker (1967) who treat aggressive behavior as relatively rare high-amplitude responses that represent a special case of a broader class of assertive behaviors. Assertive behaviors, these writers point out, have two characteristics: they demand an immediate reaction and carry the implied threat of increasingly assertive behavior in case of noncompliance. The reaction demanded from the environment very often provides reinforcing consequences, thus aiding the acquisition of these behaviors in the course of a child's socialization.

Patterson, Littman, and Bricker maintain that all children who emit aggressive behavior must previously have acquired the more general class of assertive behavior which they view as necessary, though not sufficient conditions for aggression. If assertive responses were always met by the demanded response on the part of the person to whom it is addressed, this response class would be limited to assertive behavior; that is, aggressive behavior would not develop. However, since the vagaries of human interaction do not always operate to give immediate gratification of every request, the request will often be repeated at higher intensity and, if it is then met, that higher intensity response will be the one that is strengthened and learned.

Most of the assertive behavior of young children is of relatively low amplitude and short duration because, typically, the responses are not accompanied by emotional arousal. Assertive behavior does not come to be labeled aggressive until it reaches high intensity at which point the child who emits such responses with high frequency is viewed as an aggressive child. Up to this point, this formulation is quite similar to the high-magnitude theory of aggression advanced by Bandura and Walters (1963), but Patterson, Littman, and Bricker expand on this by maintaining that *two* conditions must be met before a child is labeled as aggressive: his assertive responses must be emitted at high magnitude and frequency *and* they must be under the control of aversive motivational states which, when terminated contingent on the aggressive response, further strengthen this response. The motivational state may take several forms, including hunger, fear, or anger, and the latter may or may not be the consequence of frustration.

The theory of aggression postulated by Patterson, Littman, and Bricker thus states that two major factors are involved in the acquisition of assertive-aggressive behavior. The first entails the shaping of relevant responses into the child's repertoire by means of the reinforcers dispensed by parents, siblings, and peers. The initial training in assertive behavior is probably accomplished by the parent, but younger siblings and peers contribute to the further development of these responses. While a parent may, at least at times, insist that a yelled demand be repeated in the form of a polite request before it is granted, siblings and peers are more likely to give in when pushed, hit, or yelled at by an older sibling or stronger peer. A younger sibling can also receive training in assertive-aggressive behavior when his occasional counterassertion is reinforced, particularly in families where such behavior is encouraged or permitted by parents.

The second major factor involved in the acquisition of aggressive behavior is the high-intensity, emotional state which, when accompanying assertive-aggressive responses, makes this behavior a social problem. In order for a child to be labeled an aggressive child, he must have received massive social reinforcement for aggressive behavior, and he must also be exposed to frequent aversive emotional stimulation from his environment. Since both of these contingencies coincide relatively rarely, very few children in the general population present problems in the area of aggression. On the other hand, the two sets of contingencies may be expected to coincide more frequently in some segments of society than in others; therefore these segments would be expected to produce more children whose behavior is characterized by frequent high amplitude assertive responses that society labels as aggressive.

The insistence that an aversive motivational state be a necessary part of the definition of aggression and the statement that "very few" children present problems in the area of aggression open the Patterson, Littman, and Bricker formulation to several questions. According to this view, a child who calmly inflicts pain on an animal or who teases another child to the point of tears is not aggressive, nor would murder committed "in cold blood" be a form of aggression. To this rather idiosyncratic definition is added the surprising statement about the low frequency of aggressive problems in the general population which runs counter to the data from such surveys as that conducted by Werry and Quay (1971) and is, in fact, contradicted by the research of the Patterson group itself.

In order to test the hypothesis derived from their formulation about the acquisition of assertive-aggressive responses, Patterson, Littman, and Bricker (1967) conducted a painstaking observational study of 36 nursery school children that covered a 9-month period. During this time they recorded 2,583 aggressive responses and their consequences. Each aggressive event was coded as belonging to one of four categories: bodily attack, attack with an object, verbal or symbolic attack, and infringement of property or invasion of territory. The consequences were categorized in one of seven classes in terms of the response made by the victim of the aggression. These response consequences were passive (no response, withdrawing, or giving in), crying, assuming defensive posture, telling the teacher, recovering property, and retaliation. The seventh category, a relatively infrequent one, was teacher intervention.

On the basis of reinforcement principles it was assumed that the consequences arbitrarily labeled *positive* (passive, crying, or defensive responses on the part of the victim) would strengthen the aggressive behavior directed at that particular victim, while those consequences arbitrarily labeled *negative* (telling the teacher, recovering the property, retaliation, and teacher intervention) would weaken the aggressive behavior directed at that particular victim. In other words, it was predicted that when an assertive response was followed by a positive consequence, the aggressor would, on the next occasion, select the same aggressive response and the same victim. On the other hand, if his behavior had been followed by a negative consequence, it was predicted that he would, on the next occasion, change either the nature of the aggressive response or the victim or both.

The data supported these predictions at a high level of significance, leading to the conclusion that the typical nursery school provides social interactions that serve to maintain assertive-aggressive behavior in children. What is more, this social setting also provides an extremely efficient program for the acquisition of assertive behaviors by children who are initially passive and unassertive. These children were frequently victimized; but when they eventually counterattacked, they were reinforced by positive consequences, and after that the frequency of their initiating aggressive responses tended to increase, with this behavior showing a typical acquisition pattern.

Contrary to the investigators' expectations, the proportion of positive reinforcements a given child would provide for the aggressive behaviors of others was unrelated to the frequency with which he was victimized. Victimization did not reveal a stable pattern, but the amount of social interaction that a given child engaged in seemed to be a major factor in determining the amount and kind of reinforcement he would get for his behavior. The data reported by Patterson et al. suggest that the child who interacts with his peers at a high frequency is the one most likely to be reinforced for aggressive behavior. The highly aggressive child was found to have a high rate of peer-interaction, and the passive child with a high rate of interaction was the most likely to acquire aggressive behaviors. While peer-interaction seems to be partly a function of general activity level, the investigators believe that the child who interacts at a high rate is the child for whom peer-dispensed social reinforcers have acquired high potency. This complex interrelationship between activity level, social reinforcement, and social interaction requires further research before the relative contributions and possible causal relations of these and other factors can be known.

While the Patterson, Littman, and Bricker data lend strong support to the reinforcement formulation of the acquisition process for assertive-aggressive behavior, they recognize that not all of the subjects behaved in accordance with their theoretical predictions. Thus, there were two highly aggressive children whose behavior seems to have been maintained by other than the positive consequences dispensed by their victims, and there was one passive subject whose counterattacks were never successful but who began to acquire aggressive responses nonetheless. It appears, as the authors point out, that there are individual differences in the kind of reinforcing stimuli that control assertive responses and that no single set of generalized reinforcers for these responses applies to all children.

REDUCING AGGRESSIVE BEHAVIOR

In the discussion of their monograph, Patterson, Littman, and Bricker (1967) point to the implications of their study for the clinical treatment of children whose aggressive behavior represents a problem for their environment. Traditional treatment approaches for children with problems in this area have primarily focused on the removal of frustrations, largely on the no longer tenable assumption that frustration is the prime antecedent to aggression. Since aggression has been shown to be a response maintained by its consequences, modification of antecedent conditions will reduce the frequency of the aggression response only for as long as these antecedent conditions are kept out of the child's environment, that is, only for as long as the child remains in the highly protective institutional environment. Inasmuch as the peer group provides immediate and powerful social reinforcers that maintain aggressive behavior, the strength of this behavior will not be changed by temporary removal of the discriminative stimulus, frustration, although this can reduce the frequency of the responses for as long as this artificial condition maintains. As soon as such a child returns to the unprotected life of the community, his aggression responses will return to the pretreatment rate.

To produce more permanent changes in aggressive behavior one would have to use a dual approach aimed at weakening aggressive responses and strengthening more socially desirable behaviors to take their place. If aggressive responses are reinforced by the reactions of the peer group, one way of assuring that this reinforcement is withheld and the aggression responses placed on an extinction schedule is to remove the aggressor from his peer group immediately upon his emitting an aggression response. This principle was used successfully by Tyler and Brown (1967) who would place an offending child for 15 minutes into isolation immediately after a defined aggressive act. The fact that this "time out" procedure is not a punishment in the traditional sense but primarily a withdrawal of positive reinforcement, is illustrated by the fact that Burchard and

Tyler (1965) were thus able to reduce the antisocial behavior of a thirteen-year-old institutionalized delinquent boy who, prior to their study, had spent a total of 200 days in an individual isolation room during which time his behavior had become increasingly unmanageable. When defined acceptable behavior such as academic performance or specified time units during which no disruption occurred receives positive reinforcement, the treatment has at least a theoretical basis for success, as shown in the studies by Burchard and Tyler (1965), Tyler and Brown (1968), and Bostow and Bailey (1969).

Brown and Elliott (1965) demonstrated with a group of nursery school boys that the rate of emission of aggressive responses can be reduced through a weakening of these responses by withholding the social reinforcement and concomitantly strengthening behaviors incompatible with aggression. In that instance, the potent social reinforcer was teacher attention, and their manipulation consisted of having the teachers shift their attention from aggressive to co-operative responses. While aggressive responses among three- and four-year-old children attending a normal nursery school are apparently readily controlled by the simple manipulation of teacher attention, the operant principles involved have also been successfully applied to the disruptive behavior of children attending a third-grade adjustment class as shown by O'Leary & Becker, 1967. They introduced a token reinforcement program under which the children could earn tokens backed up by prizes for emitting defined behaviors that were incompatible with class disruption. We shall return to a discussion of these and similar treatment approaches in Chapter 14.

RECAPITULATION

In no other psychological disorder is the sociocultural relativity of the definition of what constitutes a problem quite as apparent as in the case of aggressive behavior. Depending on the circumstances, on who emits the response, and on who is the victim, the identical behavior may be called *aggression* at one time and not at another. One of the most useful definitions of aggression is a response emitted at high magnitude that society labels as aggressive. Like any other response, aggression can be learned and modified through experience with its consequences. Because of its demand characteristics which make it difficult to ignore, the aggressive response is almost invariably followed by consequences which are, often, such as to reinforce the person emitting this behavior. This is particularly true under circumstances where a response sequence is blocked before the goal is reached ("frustration"), since here an aggressive response often leads to the removal of the block, thus resulting in reinforcement. Since an aggressive response is often, some say always, accompanied by the noxious arousal state we call *anger* which is reduced with the termination of the aggressive act, this negative reinforcement is another important mode through which aggressive responses are strengthened. Once one has identified the various sources of reinforcement that maintain aggressive behavior, it is possible to modify this behavior through changing the reinforcing conditions.

10

WITHDRAWN BEHAVIOR

It may seem surprising that withdrawn behavior finds discussion under the rubric of excess behavior since, at first glance, a withdrawn child would seem to show a behavior deficit. If withdrawn behavior were the result of an absence of responses—if such a child were literally doing nothing—it would be appropriate to view withdrawn behavior as a behavior deficit. Withdrawn behavior, however, is behavior; the child is actively responding to his environment. He is not "doing nothing." His responses take the form of avoidance and escape behavior; he is actively withdrawing from contacts with his environment, and since these withdrawing responses occur in excess, the problem should be viewed as one of excess behavior. Help for such a child would have to take the form of reducing the avoidance and escape responses. Concurrently, to be sure, such a child would need help in acquiring or relearning appropriate, adaptive approach responses so that these can take the place of the maladaptive withdrawing responses.

As the word *withdrawn* suggests, these children have "drawn away" from social interactions that were at one time a part of their behavior repertoire. Children who never acquired appropriate responses for social interaction, such as those with early infantile autism, manifest a behavior deficit and are therefore not discussed in the following pages. Since age-appropriate social behavior develops gradually in the course of ongoing interactions, a child who has withdrawn from such interactions will, as he gets older, engage in behavior that is primitive and immature with respect to his chronological age. Not having age-appropriate social skills represents a deficit that is secondary to the primary excessive withdrawal; hence the need to teach him these skills as withdrawing behavior diminishes in the course of treatment.

ANXIETY

The avoidance and escape responses one observes in children whose behavior is marked by withdrawal are presumably learned under conditions where such responses reduce or eliminate aversive stimulation. An aversive stimulus, such as one associated with the sensation of pain, ordinarily elicits behavior that will result in the termination of such stimulation. Such escape behavior probably has a large innate, genetic component—its species-preserving characteristics having favored its evolution. From the standpoint of behavior economy, repeated exposure to and escape from the aversive object would be costly, and most of the time the organism, after a limited number of exposures, no longer comes face-to-face with the aversive object because he learns to avoid it. In order to explain avoidance behavior, it is necessary to postulate something that takes the place of the aversive object which, being avoided, is no longer an effective aversive stimulus. Some other aversive object or condition must mediate the avoidance behavior, something that will maintain this behavior by furnishing the reinforcing consequence otherwise rendered by the termination of the aversive stimulation of the (now avoided) object. This "something" that mediates avoidance behavior is the very useful hypothetical construct *anxiety*.

Used as a hypothetical construct, anxiety is viewed as a process that gives rise to observable phenomena, including phenomena "other than the observables that led to hypothesizing the construct" (Ruebush, 1963, p. 462). The observable phenomena which permit us to infer the presence of anxiety are measurable physiological changes, including changes in heart rate, respiratory rate, and skin conductance; changes in motor behavior, such as muscular tremors, hyperactivity, motor disorganization, and a low threshold for motor responses ("jumpiness"); and verbal reports of subjective changes, such as feelings of apprehension, worry, anticipation of threat, and sensations of fear particularly from unspecifiable sources of danger.

As used in the present context, anxiety is viewed as having physiological, motor, and cognitive components, but the identification of anxiety does not demand the demonstration of all three components in every case. It appears, in fact, that there are considerable individual differences in the way in which the three components correlate with one another (Martin, 1961). During treatment some individuals report subjective improvement and behave accordingly before changes in heart rate can be recorded, while others will show changes in heart rate before they report subjective improvement (Leitenberg et al., 1971).

Physiological Correlates of Anxiety

The basis of most of the available knowledge about the relationship between physiological changes and other measures of anxiety comes from experimental work with adults. While most theorists make the assumption that a child's experience of anxiety is accompanied by physiological changes, particularly in the autonomic system, there is little direct evidence concerning the validity of this assumption. Patterson, Helper, and Wilcott (1960) studied the relationship between anxiety and verbal conditioning in children. They used the electrical resistance of the skin (GSR) as the measure of the physiological concomitant of the anxiety which was presumably aroused in the child by having been taken to the physiological laboratory, seeing the complicated electronic equipment, having to lie down in a dimly lit room, and having electrodes taped to forearms and palms. This study emphasizes the difficulties and complexities of this type of research, for while the environmental stimuli seem to have aroused anxiety, as reflected in the children's verbalizations, the relationship between verbal conditioning and skin conductance remained ambiguous. Children with very high or very low skin conductance tended to show little conditioning, but among the high-skin-conductance children, those who inhibited motor activity acquired the conditioned verbal response (verbs on a word-association task) more rapidly than those who expressed motor activity.

A fairly simple method for assessing transitory anxiety in children, the palmar sweat print (PSP), was investigated by Lore (1966). After painting the palmar surfaces of the four fingers with a ferric chloride solution, the investigator asks the child to place his hand on a paper that has been impregnated with tannic acid. Nursery school children with an average age of 4 years and 5 months participated in Lore's study and are reported to have enjoyed the "fingerprint game." Palmar sweat dissolves the ferric chloride solution which, the latter reacting with the tannic acid, leaves a permanent stain on the paper. This stain varies in color from light gray to dark purple, and can be analyzed with a densitometer. The relative darkness or density of the print left on the paper is directly proportional to the amount of sweat secreted by the child's fingers when the print was taken. As a measure of anxiety, this method rests on the assumption that sweating is a valid indicator of the physiological changes involved in the construct "anxiety." To test this assumption, Lore read a mildly anxiety-arousing story to twelve child subjects and compared their PSP ratings with those from a control condition. He reports significant PSP score differences for group means, although for two of the twelve children the scores did not reflect an increase in anxiety.

The palmar sweat print method would seem to have interesting research potential, but since it does not permit one to take ongoing readings of physiological changes, permitting a measure at only one point in time, its applicability is somewhat limited. In order to obtain measures reflecting moment-to-moment changes in responsivity, it is still necessary to attach skin electrodes to the subject and to make polygraph recordings. The problems involved in doing this with children have limited the number of studies on the physiological correlates to anxiety in children. We must therefore refer to studies using human adults in order to discuss what changes one might expect when an individual is exposed to anxiety-arousing stimuli.

Most relevant to the findings of Lore (1966) and of Patterson et al. (1960), which were cited above, is the pioneering work by Ax (1953) who exposed adults to a condition designed to arouse fear and another condition designed to arouse anger and found that skin conductance increased under both conditions. Increases in skin conductance thus cannot be viewed as unequivocal evidence of anxiety. Different physiological measures do, however, permit one to assess anxiety and to differentiate this hypothetical state from the hypothetical state of anger. Thus it appears that diastolic blood pressure increases more for anger than for anxiety and that heart rate increases more in fear than in anger. A fairly readily available observation that could be used in work with children is that the mucosa of the nose appear to show a blanching in anxiety and an engorgement and redness in anger (Martin, 1961).

On the endocrine level one finds fairly convincing research data that point to a relationship between secretions from the adrenal medulla and reports of anxiety and anger. According to these data (Ax, 1953) epinephrine (adrenalin) produces a rise in systolic blood pressure, in pulse rate, and in stroke volume, that is, an increased cardiac output with concomitant vasodilation. Subjects manifesting these changes generally verbalize subjective anxiety, and the autonomic pattern described has come to be labeled an "epinephrinelike" reaction (Funkenstein, King, & Drolette, 1957). This reaction appears to be distinctly different from the "norepinephrinelike" pattern—the primary feature of which is vasoconstriction, accompanied by a rise in diastolic blood pressure and a fall in pulse rate and stroke volume. This reaction is often accompanied by expressions of anger, provided such anger is directed outward. Individuals whose tendency is to turn their anger inward, verbalizing self-blame and guilt, are reported to show the "epinephrinelike" pattern upon biochemical analysis.

Funkenstein, King, and Drolette (1957) differentiate between three major emotional reaction patterns—anger directed outward, anger directed inward, and fear and/or anxiety. As pointed out, they report that the physiological concomitants of anger directed outward is the excessive secretion of a norepinephrinelike substance, while anger directed inward and anxiety are accompanied by physiological evidence of excessive secretion of an epinephrinelike substance. Discussing psychological and physiological development these authors refer to evidence that "anger-out" is characteristic of an earlier period of development than "anger-in" or "severe-anxiety," a reaction where anxiety is dominant over emotional components. According to this view it is only in the course of socialization that the child learns to turn anger inward or to react to certain stimuli with anxiety. Funkenstein, King, and Drolette (1957) state:

> Since Anger-Out was found to be associated with nor-epinephrine, and Anger-In and Severe-Anxiety with epineph-rine in adults, it would be expected that, since Anger-Out represents a reaction characteristic of an earlier stage of development, the adrenal medulla at birth and in early infancy would contain predominately nor-epinephrine and that as the child developed epinephrine would then be secreted [p. 171].

These authors cite findings from physiological studies showing that at birth the adrenal gland indeed contains predominantly noradrenalin (norepinephrine), while adrenalin (epinephrine) is gradually added as the child develops, eventually becoming the dominant adrenal secretion. Thus, Hökfelt (1951) reported that the adrenal gland of the human fetus at the end of 3 months contains no adrenaline but 1 microgram of noradrenaline. Six weeks later, 3 micrograms of adrenaline and 25 micrograms of noradrenaline were isolated. In children under 70 days of age, adrenal output is 90 percent noradrenaline (Shepherd & West, 1951), while in the two-year-old child adrenaline has become dominant, representing 60 percent of the hormone output of the adrenal. Finally, in the human adult, the balance is 80 percent adrenaline and 20 percent noradrenaline (Hökfelt, 1951). These findings led Shepherd and West (1951) to the speculation that in the early stage of human life the need for epinephrine is very small.

If these research results are valid and the speculations justified they would have important theoretical implications inasmuch as they suggest that the infant lacks the physiological capacity for an anxiety response. The learning of fear responses to specific classes of environmental stimuli and their generalization (anxiety) thus could not take place until at least several months after birth, and even then the reaction would be less pronounced than in the adult.

While there appear to be hormonal differences in anger and in anxiety, it is important to note that the relevant studies report large individual differences both in terms of the intensity of the reaction and in the nature of the reaction. Thus, Schachter (1957) found epinephrinelike responses in an anxiety-arousing situation, norepinephrinelike patterns following the application of a painful stimulus, but mixed patterns when anger was aroused. Here some subjects reacted in the epinephrinelike pattern, others in the norepinephrinelike pattern, while a few displayed a combined pattern. One might speculate that some of the subjects in this experiment had, in previous life situations, learned to react to their own anger with anxiety, but the fact that in Schachter's experiment the fear-arousal phase preceded the anger-arousal phase and the same experimenter who had been instrumental in arousing the fear also aroused the anger may have introduced stimulus generalization and thus confounded the data.

The difficulty in relating a physiological arousal state to a subjectively reported emotion was demonstrated in the frequently cited experiment by Schachter and Singer (1962) which showed that how a subject will label his arousal depends on the situation in which he finds himself at the time. These investigators hypothesized that when a subject has no ready explanation for the source of his arousal, he labels it in terms of the information available to him at the time. Some subjects in this experiment received an injection of adrenalin under the guise of studying the effects of a vitamin supplement. Adrenalin is known to result in increased systolic blood pressure, heart rate, respiration, blood flow to muscles and brain, and a decreased blood flow to the skin. The subjective experience of these changes and the concomitant increases in blood sugar and lactic acid concentration are palpitation, tremor, and, for some individuals, a feeling of accelerated breathing and flushing. After receiving information regarding the effect to be expected from this injection (which differed depending on the group to which the subject had been assigned), each subject was placed with another who was in reality a confederate of the experimenters. With half the subjects this confederate behaved angrily, while with the other half he behaved euphorically. The results clearly indicated that the subjects who had not been given an explanation for the changes in their sensations were highly susceptible to the apparent mood of the confederate, both in terms of how they behaved and in terms of the feelings they reported experiencing.

The Development of the Fear Response

In a review of certain features of infant-mother relationship in mammals and birds, King (1966) postulates that one important basis for the infant's attraction to the mother is the fear-reducing capacity of some aspects of the stimulus configuration of the mother. He suggests that the mother or a component of her is a stimulus that innately elicits a response ("pleasure") which is incompatible with and hence reducing of fear. King interprets available research as indicating that novel stimuli are innately fear-eliciting without their having to be painful or associated with pain in the past. He states that stimuli will elicit fear depending on their degree of novelty. Accordingly, familiar objects in an unfamiliar position or setting or stimuli in constantly changing movement are conceived as containing novel elements, and sudden changes in stimulus pattern, such as a loud noise in a normally quiet environment, would also be novel.

These hypotheses lead to the dilemma that they would predict an infant to react with fear to the mother, for she would be a novel stimulus not only when first encountered but also each time she is encountered in different conditions and environments. This issue can be resolved if one postulates that fear of novel stimuli is a maturational phenomenon. King (1966) suggests that the infant does not respond with fear to first exposure to his mother—a novel stimulus—because there is a period after birth in which novel stimuli do not have the capacity to elicit fear responses, and the ability of novel stimuli to elicit fear develops gradually as maturation progresses. Hormonal studies previously cited suggest that the reason novel stimuli do not elicit fear responses in very young infants is that they have not yet developed the physiological capacity to respond with fear and that this capacity develops gradually as epinephrine output increases with age.

By the time the infant reaches the developmental stage where he is capable of fear responses so that novel stimuli can elicit fear, the "pleasure" response elicited by the stimulus configuration "mother" has become firmly established, and as a result of the strength of this response and the initial weakness of the fear response, the fear-incompatible "pleasure" response is stronger whenever a novel stimulus is encountered in the presence of his mother. Such a state of affairs would result in the highly adaptive capacity of the infant to encounter and explore novel stimuli *provided* he is in the presence of his mother. Once these stimuli have been encountered under these conditions, they will gradually cease to be novel and become familiar and eventually no longer fear-eliciting but pleasure-eliciting. On the other hand, if the infant encounters a novel stimulus when his mother is not present, this analysis would predict that he should respond with fear and avoidance behavior that should result in his returning to the mother in whose presence fear is reduced by the incompatible "pleasure" response. This being the case, the mother should eventually acquire secondary reinforcement value, being not only the "pleasure" elicitor (a capacity she may well lose after a certain maturational period) but also the fear-reducer. If one adds to these considerations the mother's other reinforcement dispensing activities, the young child's tendency to remain near and return to her and to show distress when she is absent can be readily understood. This formulation also suggests an explanation for the fact that young children frequently share their mothers' fears. If novel stimuli lose their fear-arousing capacity when they are encountered in the presence of the mother, those stimuli which the mother avoids because of her own fears could not be encountered in the mother's presence and would thus remain potentially novel and fear-arousing for the child.

While King (1966) suggests that the fear-eliciting function of novel stimuli develops as a maturational phenomenon, it seems necessary to ask whether this function also declines after a certain developmental phase. In other words, is there a critical period during which novel stimuli elicit fear? The reason for this question is the well-supported observation that human children and mammals engage in exploratory behavior and that they show a preference for novel stimuli when given a choice under certain conditions (Berlyne,

1960). This preference would not be found if novel stimuli were fear-eliciting throughout the developmental span. Hunt (1961), in reviewing the development of intelligence and its relationship to experience, suggests that curiosity does not develop until Piaget's developmental stage of tertiary circular reactions, that is, not until the child is at about the end of his first year of life. He points out that the child's discovery of the movements and changes he can produce in objects he manipulates brings about an interest in novelty which, in turn, gives rise to curiosity, that is, the behavior manifested in preference for novelty. This would suggest that the critical period during which novel stimuli have the capacity to elicit fear comes to a gradual end around the beginning of the second year of life. The beginning of this critical period may well be around 6 months, for while hormonal studies do not provide a clue to this, the frequently reported fear of strangers that appears around that age would suggest that then the infant is becoming capable of discriminating novel stimuli and of responding to them with fear.

While fear with its identifiable physiological correlates may not occur until some months after birth, more primitive forms of distress appear present from the earliest days of a child's life. Traditionally, it has been assumed that fear is the unconditioned response to the unconditioned stimulus of pain and that all further elicitation of fear or of its generalized form, anxiety, is based on the classical conditioning paradigm, whereby a neutral (conditioned) stimulus is paired with the presentation of pain and thus comes to acquire fear-eliciting capacity in its own right.

The limitation of this traditional assumption is apparent when one recalls that a newborn infant will display marked signs of distress when he is exposed to sudden loss of physical support, a condition not previously paired with pain. To reconcile this paradox, Kessen and Mandler (1961) suggest the concept of "fundamental distress" as a condition that has a cyclical appearance in the human newborn and for which no antecedent event need be postulated. They further propose that certain events in the environment and responses of the organism serve as specific inhibitors of distress, naming nonnutritive sucking, rocking, and rhythmical stimulation as among these inhibitors. When other, previously neutral, events are paired with the presentation of a specific inhibitor, these events will become secondary inhibitors through the mechanism of conditioning. This formulation, though highly speculative, permits one to perceive the development of fear responses under conditions not involving the infliction of pain.

From the standpoint of a discussion of psychological disorders it is of little import to ask how anxiety originally came to be a part of a child's behavior repertoire. The facts appear to be the following: certain situations, different for different children, have the capacity to elicit the arousal response we call anxiety; this response (anxiety) has noxious qualities; and other responses that are followed by a reduction of anxiety tend to be strengthened. When these responses are maladaptive because they interfere with the child's expected life role, they and the anxiety which maintains them become problems calling for alleviation. The fact that procedures based on the principles of learning can be used to reduce the anxiety and, hence, the associated avoidance responses is strongly suggestive of the hypothesis that these principles were also operating when anxiety was acquired but there is little evidence that this was indeed the case. The frequently cited demonstration of a learned fear response, reported by Watson and Raynor (1920) in the classical case of Albert, shows only that a fear response can be learned, but this study cannot be used to support the contention that all fear responses are learned nor that the fear responses of a specific child seen in a clinical situation were originally acquired through learning.

The Limitations of Verbal Reports

Recordings of physiological arousal states give the appearance of great objectivity because they are represented in the form of mechanically produced tracing on paper tape. Unfortunately, the intercorrelation of various physiological measures is so low and the individual differences in reactivity are so high that these measures have little clinical utility in the present state of knowledge and technique. For this reason and because it is far easier to ask a child questions than to attach electrodes to his body, most research on anxiety in children has taken the form of questionnaire studies.

Most of these studies start from the premise that anxiety is a state, an enduring though fluctuating condition in which the child finds himself at all times and which can be measured without reference to environmental circumstances. If one construes anxiety as a response, learned to and elicited by specific situations and possibly generalized from these, the research literature on anxiety-as-a-state has limited relevance.

Research on anxiety-as-a-response requires that one present the child with a stressful stimulus (or study him in a naturally occurring crisis situation) and measure his anxiety. The methodological and ethical difficulties in conducting such research are readily apparent. One cannot expose a child to truly stressful situations merely for the sake of studying his reactions. The moment one uses some attenuated stress one does not know whether the stimulus is anxiety-arousing, for to ascertain this one would need a measure that is independent of the one to be used in the study. Moreover, stressful stimuli are usually transitory, yet anxiety questionnaires take time to administer. For these reasons, negative results are impossible to interpret. They may mean that no anxiety was elicited because the stimulus was not anxiety-arousing. Or they may mean that the stimulus was anxiety-arousing but that the subject did not respond with anxiety. Or they may mean that the stimulus was anxiety-arousing and that the subject responded with anxiety but that his anxiety had dissipated by the time the questionnaire was administered. Then again, the questionnaire might not have been a valid measure of anxiety—or a combination of all these factors was at play. With all these problems, it is not surprising that experimental anxiety studies using verbal reports as a measure have failed to obtain significant results (Ruebush, 1963).

The current state of research-based knowledge about anxiety in children is thus one of considerable ignorance. We have a widely used hypothetical construct which can be defined in terms of observable phenomena. We know that changes in endocrine secretion are correlated with certain changes in physiological state but that verbal labels of these subjectively experienced changes are unreliable. Developmental issues are barely explored and a practical methodology for studying anxiety responses through self-report has yet to be developed. Despite all that, the hypothetical construct *anxiety* serves such an important heuristic function that a discussion of behavior disorders is virtually impossible without recourse to this construct.

ANXIETY AND DISTURBED BEHAVIOR

As will be seen in the following, some behavior disorders are maintained by the anxiety-reducing consequences of the child's maladaptive responses. Since the behavior can thus be construed as disturbed by the emotion of anxiety, the term *emotionally disturbed* might be used appropriately in these cases. This term has unfortunately been used so loosely that it has lost its original meaning and serves largely to confuse the issue. In fields such as special education the expression emotionally disturbed has come to cover every form of behavior disorder, including the most profound impairments. Since there is no evidence that an emotion is implicated in every form of disturbed behavior, it seems best to restrict the use of *emotional disturbance* to those cases where behavior problems can be demonstrated to be the direct consequence of an emotion, such as generalized fear. Even in those cases it should be kept in mind that the emotion is disturbing the behavior and that it is not the emotion that is disturbed, as the term emotionally disturbed would tend to suggest.

Children who emit a high rate of avoidance responses to a wide variety of situations will tend to avoid social interactions and thus have few friends and limited interests. Their behavior is generally maintained on a very low rate of positive reinforcement, and they typically exhibit frequent crying spells, marked sensitivity to criticism, easy discouragement in the face of failure, extensive worry, lack of enthusiasm and interest, and a generalized sad and listless approach to tasks. These characteristics have led such children to be labeled *depressed,* but it is doubtful that this label contributes anything to the understanding of their problem. Like all other terms that involve an inference about a child's internal state, *depression* must be translated into operational terms that refer to observable behavior before one can hope to do something constructive for the child. When a child encounters few positive reinforcements, one would want to expose him to situations that provide opportunities for experiencing positive consequences for adaptive behavior. Often that means that he has to be taught age-appropriate skills, including social skills, before he can make use of such opportunities. At the same time, one must not overlook the fact that the child's withdrawn behavior is a function of excessive avoidance responses. Since these avoidance responses must be recognized and reduced if the child is to learn adaptive approach responses, it is to these avoidance responses that we now turn our attention.

Fears and Phobias

Realistic fears have survival value; hence all children should have some fear of potentially dangerous objects or situations. Fears create problems when they are excessive or attached to stimuli that are not objectively dangerous. When a specific fear is so strong that it interferes with the child's ability to function adaptively, it is usually called a *phobia*, and, depending on its object, one can speak of dog phobia, bee phobia, snake phobia, etc. Since any neutral stimulus can acquire phobia-eliciting characteristics, the list is without limit. Some children come to be afraid of losing a parent by death or abandonment and find that they can reduce the fear by staying close to that parent, not letting him out of sight. This *separation anxiety* will prevent the child from attending school, but it should not be confused with school phobia, an excessive and disabling fear of school that leads to the avoidance of school, not the avoidance of leaving the parent. Other children may be afraid of illness, injury, or death; and, like other fears, these may be elaborated in fantasy, so that darkness, being left alone, new situations, or unexpected changes may come to acquire fear-arousing properties.

The problem characterized by strong fears associated with attending school and verbalizations of vague dread and apprehensions about disaster is usually called *school phobia.* In these cases, the child frequently complains about such physical problems as headaches, stomachaches, or nausea. It is not unusual for such children to express additional fears about a variety of things, such as darkness or being left alone.

Kennedy (1965) differentiated between two types of school phobia. Type 1 is characterized by an acute onset representing the first such episode in a child who is in his early years of school. The problem often occurs on a Monday, following brief illness and authorized absence from school the previous week. The child often expresses concern about death and about his mother's physical health. His parents' psychological state is usually unremarkable, and they are in good communication with one another. They share responsibility for family management and respond to efforts at helping their child with understanding and cooperation. Kennedy's Type 2, on the other hand, characterizes cases where school refusal has occurred several times before and where the original onset was gradual. It occurs mostly in the upper grades and can start on any day of the week. In these cases, the parents have poor communication and manifest psychological or behavior problems of their own. The father tends to show little interest in household or children, and the parents fail to cooperate in the treatment procedures aimed at getting their child back to school.

It is very likely that school phobia represents an overdetermined response pattern. Nearly all children, at one time or another, express a reluctance to go to school. If the parent deals with this reluctance in a matter-of-fact way and insists that school attendance is expected and required, nothing will come of the incident. On the other hand, if the parent begins to make lengthy inquiries into why the child does not want to go to school, eliciting more or less plausible and more or less factual rationalizations, and then agrees to let the child stay home, the basis of future school avoiding behavior may well be laid. For other children, an event or series of events at school have a highly noxious quality, making school, in fact, a fear-arousing situation. Being teased or attacked by other children, losing in competition, fighting with a friend, or being embarrassed by the need for physical exposure in connection with undressing for gym may all initiate fear of school and school refusal. Some of the circumstances just listed may be more critical for girls than for boys, and this may account for the fact that school refusal is one of the few forms of psychological disorder for which boys do not outnumber girls; for here the incidence among girls is at least as great as among boys, some reports actually pointing to a higher incidence for girls (Talbot, 1957).

Once a child refuses to go to school, thus avoiding the fear-arousing conditions he would encounter there, remaining at home and the reinforcing qualities this entails will lend secondary support to the avoidance behavior. Being allowed to watch television, being fed by mother, having people fuss over you because you are "sick" will all conspire to make it more difficult for the child to return to school. What is more, once several days of school have been missed, returning there becomes ever more unpleasant to contemplate. The child will have missed instructional content and thus find himself behind the rest of the class with the aversive consequences this implies. Also, returning after an absence often results in being singled out for curious attention and questions about the reason for the absence which, in this case, are embarrassing to answer. In fact, returning to school after a few days of absence due to physical illness is unpleasant for many children, and, as in Kennedy's Type 1, it is not unusual for school refusals to have their onset immediately after such legitimate absence, including, at times, a long weekend.

Lazarus, Davison, and Polefka (1965) took cognizance of the multiple factors that maintain a school phobia by treating a nine-year-old boy using both respondent and operant formulations and procedures. They reduced the intense fear of school by the therapeutic procedure called *systematic desensitization* and then limited as many as possible of the reinforcements for staying at home. At the same time, they began to reward school-approaching behavior, thus, in effect, reversing the contingencies; where school-avoiding behavior had received reinforcing attention, such attention was now focused on its reciprocal—school-approaching behavior. Cooperation from the school permitted a variety of modifications in their routine; thus the boy's reentry problem was eased.

Because school refusal is strengthened by the reinforcing events encountered while away from school, it has been recognized that this behavior must be reversed as soon as possible after onset if intervention is to be successful. Giving a child spurious medical excuses and facilitating instruction at home until he "gets over" his problem are by now generally recognized as achieving exactly the opposite of what is intended—to get the child back to school. Kennedy (1965) stressed the need for immediate intervention, starting as soon as the child refuses to go to school. The treatment approach he advocates for his Type 1 cases calls for intervention on the second or third day after onset of the problem. Avoiding emphasis on somatic complaints, the therapist is firm in his insistence on school attendance, even to the point of using force if necessary. An interview with the parents helps them take an active part in the treatment plan which has its focus on reinforcing school attendance and reducing the reinforcing value of sympathy, or concern about his "condition." Following this approach, Kennedy reported success in all of his fifty cases, and follow-up, lasting in some instances over 8 years, revealed neither a repetition of school refusal nor "any outbreaks of substitute symptoms" (p. 287).

While forced exposure to the feared situation, together with reinforcement of approach behavior, seems successful in overcoming acute school phobia problems which have had little opportunity to become confounded by various secondary gains, the chronic and complex Type 2 cases seem to call for treatment of more than school refusal. Kennedy's description of his Type 2 cases suggests, in fact, that for them school refusal was only one of a variety of other problems, including family disorganization, antisocial behavior, and profound psychological disorders requiring institutionalization. Kennedy, and others, find these cases very difficult to treat.

One of the reasons why immediate intervention and early return to school are so important in cases of school refusal is that missing instructional content makes resumption of studies more difficult, and hence, return to school more aversive. Whenever a child's schooling has been interrupted or his learning ability impaired for any length of time, help calls for reducing the behavior that is incompatible with school attendance and learning, accompanied by simultaneous efforts to strengthen learning-appropriate behavior. In addition, and because of the cumulative nature of education, these children need the benefits of intensive remedial educational efforts, designed to help them catch up with all the basic skills they failed to acquire during the time their learning disorder interfered with their acquisition of knowledge and skills. Unless such a child can be helped to reach his age-appropriate achievement level, the school experience will continue to be unrewarding, and he is likely to resume making avoidance responses to school and learning.

RECAPITULATION

The relative brevity of this chapter reflects the paucity of research dealing with avoidance behavior of children. For readily apparent reasons it is very difficult to undertake laboratory studies of children's fear and anxiety. Thus, much of what is known in this area is based on research with adult volunteers or with animals. Despite this dearth of sound knowledge about anxiety, it is next to impossible to discuss psychological disorders without reference to the construct anxiety. A discussion of school avoidance was used to illustrate the role of fear in avoidance learning and the therapeutic implications of such a formulation. More extreme forms of withdrawn behavior which can take on psychotic proportions are discussed in the following chapter.

11

DISORDERS OF PSYCHOTIC DIMENSIONS

Withdrawn behavior can range on a dimension of severity from mild to profound, from the child who is socially shy in specific situations to the one whose total relationship to other people is grossly distorted and disrupted. The words describing these severely impaired children are imprecise, and there is no agreement on terminology. Frequent and authoritative usage to the contrary (Kessler, 1966; Goldfarb, 1970), there is no evidence to support the notion that *childhood psychosis* is any more than a term loosely used to label a vaguely circumscribed cluster of severely disordered behaviors. For this reason it seems best to use *psychotic* in its adjectival form, denoting no more than a profound level of disorder. Several other terms have been used to describe profoundly disturbed children. Among these are *childhood schizophrenia* (Bender, 1947), *atypical children* (e.g., Brown, 1960), and *autistic* and *symbiotic infantile psychosis* (Mahler, 1952). Some writers (e.g., Kessler, 1966) consider childhood schizophrenia as a subcategory of childhood psychosis; others (e.g., Goldfarb, 1970) seem to consider the two to be synonymous. Little can be gained at this point from joining the issue and debating whether schizophrenia and psychosis are or are not the same "thing." In all likelihood they are not "things" or distinct entities but words that have been used to label children who display certain clusters of profoundly disturbed behavior. We shall, therefore, look at this behavior and not bother with "diagnostic" niceties, other than to have singled out *early infantile autism* for separate discussion (Chapter 4) since such a differentiation appears to have some heuristic merit.

When a child becomes profoundly withdrawn after an initial period of unremarkable development, his problem differs from that of the child who manifested deviant behavior from the beginning of life. It is this difference in onset that would seem to argue that the first instance represents a behavioral excess where the withdrawal is "added" to the child's response repertoire. In the latter instance, on the other hand, interpersonal contact has never developed; therefore one is justified in speaking of a behavior deficit. Rimland (1964) has pointed out that the time of onset is one of the criteria by which childhood schizophrenia can be differentiated from early infantile autism, and following his lead, we have presented autism in the context of other behavior deficits.

Children with psychotic disorders, including childhood schizophrenia, tend to be withdrawn, aloof, distant, and uninvolved with people, although an extreme clinging to one person (usually the mother) to the exclusion of other contacts can be observed in some instances. When the mother of such a clinging child in turn focuses her attention almost exclusively on that child, the relationship has been called *symbiotic*, implying that the two sustain each other's behavior by reciprocal reinforcement.

PSYCHOTIC DISORDERS

Despite differences in terminology, careful observers of children with psychotic disorders agree on a series of characteristics which many of these children have in common. Goldfarb (1970), citing the work of a British committee of psychiatrists, lists nine such "schizophrenic" characteristics. These are

1. Distorted interpersonal relationships, including aloofness and withdrawal

2. Disorientation with respect to the child's own person and body in relation to the environment, including self-injurious and bizarre explorations of his body

3. Bizarre preoccupation with specific objects without regard to their accepted function

4. Demand for sameness in the environment and a concomitant resistance to change

5. Atypical responses to sensory stimuli, such as apparent insensitivity to pain or excessive responses to stimulation

6. Distorted and excessive fears in the absence of objective danger with a concomitant absence of fear in the face of real danger

7. Use of speech to communicate bizarre and meaningless content; absence of or greatly immature language

8. Poor coordination, locomotion, and balance; body whirling and toe-walking; and excessive motility, immobility, bizarre posturing, or rocking

9. Extensive retardation with occasional "islands" of normal or near normal intellectual function.

This list is presented in order to give an impression of the pervasive nature of psychotic disorders. Clearly, not all children with psychotic disorders will manifest all these problems, and at least two of them—preservation of sameness and language disturbance—will be recognized as among the defining characteristics of early infantile autism. The list should therefore not be used to attempt a differentiation among children with profound psychological disorders.

The variability among children with psychotic disorders is reflected in a paper by Brown (1960) who reports that among 40 children with "atypical development," 21 had some language, 36 showed low frustration tolerance, 26 had strong or unusual years, while 20 displayed primitive object manipulation or diffuse aggression.

The following description of a "schizophrenic child" seen by this writer (Ross, 1955) places many of these behavioral aberrations in context:

The boy was brought to the clinic at age 5 years, 11 months, when his mother sought help because the child embarrassed her by his peculiar behavior, and because of certain purposeless movements of the upper extremities. She stated that there was something definitely wrong with him because he did not act like other children his age. She mentioned his fondness for examining women's purses, his running into rest rooms looking under commodes to explore the pipes, his getting on his knees to examine women's legs, and his desire to rub his hands over the hair of other children and then smelling his hands. Because of these actions, as well as a tendency to strike other children on the head, the mother stated that he "needs watching all the time." She added that the boy prefers to remain at home and to play by himself. When he occasionally joins other children, the shooting of a cap pistol creates intense fear in him. In playing hide-and-go-seek, he screams when the other child comes out of hiding and when it is his turn to hide, he insists that his mother accompany him.

During subsequent interviews with the mother further "strange behavior" was reported. The boy likes to listen to the radio and seems to prefer popular music with a pronounced rhythm. He is extremely preoccupied with the daily mail delivery and will ask constantly whether the mail has come and accosts the mailman when he arrives at the house. Fender aprons of trucks are of particular fascination to him and he will crawl under trucks to examine them. He calls these aprons "rainwater" and when he sees a vehicle without them, he'll get upset and cry, "Put the rainwater on, Mommy, put the rainwater on."

The mother dated the onset of the child's difficulties as occurring when he was two years old, although at another time she claimed that she first noticed something strange about the time a younger brother was born when the boy was one year old. As an infant, he was said to have shown anticipatory posture at feeding, reaching out for bottle and mother. He was friendly, would coo and look at everybody and notice everything so that the parents thought that he was a bright baby. His first smile is dated as occurring at three months; he took his first unassisted step around one year of age but had some difficulty in this area, and when seen at the clinic was wearing corrective shoes because of his "habit of walking on his toes." The child began to utter single words before he was 13 months old, and spoke in short sentences by two years although his speech remains difficult to understand even at this time, in part, because he has a high-pitched, squealy voice.

During a 20 minute interview with the boy he showed no evidence of any interpersonal contact. He ignored the psychiatrist and played oblivious to all distractions and external stimuli. He put strange objects into his mouth and evidently explored them in this way rather than by looking or with his hands. He was rather clumsy but there was no gross disturbance of motor behavior. Whenever he became excited, which was rather frequently, he would jump up and down and move his arms in a rapid, apparently purposeless, repetitive movement. He whirled about several times whenever his body was turned by the doctor. On two or three occasions, he became interested in the doctor's foot or hand if one of these was placed directly in front of him, but there was no evidence that he recognized it as a part of someone else's body.

This boy thus displayed each of the behavioral characteristics considered typical of the "schizophrenic syndrome" by the group cited in Goldfarb's (1970) review. The child's use of language is particularly noteworthy since, unlike most children with early infantile autism, he had developed speech but used it to communicate bizarre content, such as the references to "rainwater." Again, unlike the case of early infantile autism, this boy was aware of his environment but was confused, disoriented, and anxious about it as in his concern about the mail delivery. His strong fears and hypersensitivity to noise are further characteristics of a schizophrenic child, as are his toe walking, whirling, and repetitive behaviors.

Little is known about the factors causing schizophrenic disorders, but available information strongly suggests that one is dealing here with a behavior cluster to which an impairment of central nervous system functions makes a significant contribution. Thus, while the specific fears and preoccupations are undoubtedly learned response patterns, the overreaction and inability to cope with the fears may very well be a function of a biological predisposition. An ambitious longitudinal study by Mednick and Schulsinger (1968) promises to throw some light on this topic. Assuming that children born of schizophrenic mothers have a high risk of becoming psychiatric casualties, these investigators examined 207 such children in 1962–1963. At the time these children were functioning normally. Data on 104 children of normal mothers were gathered for purposes of control and with the intention of following these 311 children for the next 20 to 25 years. It was estimated that during that period approximately 100 of the high-risk children would develop a psychological disorder, about 30 of these being diagnosed as schizophrenic.

When the project reached its sixth year, Mednick (1970) reported that twenty of the children of schizophrenic mothers had suffered severe psychiatric breakdown. An analysis of the data from the earlier assessment made it possible to identify a number of premorbid characteristics which distinguished these subjects from the controls. Two of the most clearly discriminating characteristics were (1) the presence of a poorly controlled, hyperresponsive autonomic nervous system as measured by a physiological conditioning-generalization-extinction test and (2) history of pregnancy and delivery complications at time of birth. Since the association between these complications and the autonomic hyperresponsiveness was absent in the control group, Mednick (1970) speculates that birth complications trigger some characteristic which may be genetically predisposed. He suggests that these complications damage the modulatory control of the body's stress-response mechanism such that in an autonomic conditioning experiment the subject will display rapid response onset, poor habituation of the response, poor extinction, and very rapid recovery from the response. A review of various animal studies led Mednick to the hypothesis that the pregnancy and delivery complications result in damage to the hippocampus, an important inhibitory center of the brain. Defective hippocampal functioning "in combination with genetic and environmental factors could conceivably play a vital predispositional role in at least some forms of schizophrenia" (ibid., p. 59). This carefully worded hypothesis is in line with Mednick's theoretical orientation, for he views schizophrenia as a pattern of well-learned avoidance responses. A defective stress-response mechanism might well increase avoidance responses, and the rapid recovery from stress which is typical of hippocampal lesions would occasion immediate reinforcement of this response.

While Mednick's formulation must await further data from his impressive study, other research points in the same direction. Thus, Goldfarb (1970) concluded from an extensive review of available studies on various psychotic disorders of children that "the accumulated data . . . provide rather indisputable evidence of impairment of the central nervous system" (p. 804), though he hastens to add that this evidence is not found in all the children diagnosed as psychotic.

The Putative Role of the Mother

It is a common clinical observation that mothers of children called *schizophrenic* are tense, anxious, and preoccupied with their child's problem. This has led some to the totally unwarranted conclusion that the mother's behavior is the sole cause of the child's disturbance. The term *schizophrenogenic mother* was coined to lend credence to this logical fallacy that leaps from an observed correlation of two variables to the conclusion that one of these variables is the cause of the other. It should be apparent from the description of a psychotic disorder given above that the task of coping with such a severely disturbed child is likely to be a strain that will be reflected in the behavior of most mothers. The explanation that the child's condition causes the mother's psychological state is thus as logical, though no more warranted, as the obverse conclusion. Until data based on careful research permit a more conclusive statement, it is best to limit etiological speculations to the hypothesis that childhood schizophrenia and related psychotic disorders of children result from an interaction of several factors—some constitutional, some environmental. Such a multifactor hypothesis of the development of psychotic disorders of children would view a given child's behavior as the product of the influences of his constitutional defects and of the reaction pattern of his social environment (Ross, 1964b). Both of these factors, as Goldfarb (1970) has observed, can vary in their degree of deviation from the expected so that their relative contribution to the child's behavior disorder will vary along a continuum.

As pointed out in the beginning of this discussion, there is considerable terminological confusion and a lack of agreement on definition in the general area of psychotic disorders of children. This has greatly handicapped definitive research in this area; and it is not surprising that few studies report the same results, for different investigators have included different clusters of behavior under the loose rubrics of childhood psychosis, childhood schizophrenia, or children with atypical development.

By the time a child with a psychotic disorder becomes a subject in a study, he has passed through a number of selective screens. First, one of his parents must recognize that his behavior is deviant and become concerned about this. Usually, both parents have to agree that something is wrong before they will seek professional advice. The first such adviser is usually not a specialist in psychological disorders but a general practitioner or pediatrician. Depending on his level of sophistication, the parents may be told that "nothing is wrong, he will grow out of it," or they may be referred to any variety of specialists for audiologic, neurologic, or metabolic evaluations. An unknown proportion of children whom others might label psychotic or schizophrenic are probably being treated as if they were deaf, mentally retarded, or brain damaged. It is usually only after many other diagnostic possibilities have been ruled out that some specialist will eventually suggest psychiatric help, and even at this point, the child may be given a variety of diagnostic labels other than the one under which he will become a subject in someone's research on schizophrenic or psychotic children. At each of these dispositional choice-points, the parents' level of education and economic status contribute to the outcome because these determine both the kind of help they will seek and the kind of help they will get. Given these sources of sampling bias, any statements about "parents of schizophrenic children" is bound to be a gross overgeneralization. Until a large-scale, epidemiologic study is conducted that applies a uniform nomenclature to a population-wide survey, little, if anything, will be known about the relationship of family background to psychological disorders of children. People who bring their child to any one kind of clinic or institution are not representative of all parents of disturbed children. The following discussion should be read in light of these qualifications.

Research on Parental Behavior

The question of the etiology of psychotic disorders of children has attracted a number of investigators who have addressed themselves to the hypothesis that parental behavior is a factor in the development of the child's disturbance. The usual research strategy is to compare a group of parents of severely disturbed children with parents of normal or physically impaired controls. Thus, Bindman (1966) assessed the interaction of the parents of three groups of males: early childhood schizophrenics, young adult schizophrenics with poor adjustment, and college freshmen. He found that in both groups of schizophrenics the mothers were superior to their spouses on a conceptual sorting task, that they dominated verbal interaction with their husbands, and that they masked or denied conflict with their husbands in a discussion of child-rearing problems. Bindman also reports that the parents of the childhood schizophrenics were of a higher social class than the normals, while the parents of the adult schizophrenics came from the lower class. These findings of social class differences stand in marked contrast to a report by McDermott et al. (1967) who found no significant differences in the incidence of psychosis in children among five social class groups, suggesting that Bindman's results may be due to sampling bias or unreliable diagnostic labeling.

Speculations about maternal behavior or family environment as causal factors in childhood schizophrenia and similar psychotic disorders must invariably answer the question why these severely disturbed children have normal siblings who are, after all, raised by the same mother and in a similar environment. Sloat (1966) addressed a study to this issue by seeking to compare the child-rearing practices experienced by a group of schizophrenic children with those experienced by their nonpsychotic siblings. Her data were based on interviews conducted with 10 families in which there was a schizophrenic child and at least 1 normal sibling, both of whom were between the ages of five and twelve. Using interview schedules based on previous work on child rearing, such as that of Bandura and Walters (1959), she had 2 independent judges rate child-rearing practices and parental attitudes. The questions specifically investigated were whether there were differences in the amount of time the children had been separated from the parents, in early training procedures, in physical health, in how they were disciplined, in how their aggression was dealt with, in how early sexual behavior had been handled, or in how protected they had been. In none of these areas were there any drastic differences, although there were some suggestions that the schizophrenic children had been less accepted as infants, handled less, and talked to less at the age of acquiring speech. Sloat speculated that this may have been because these children did not respond satisfyingly and that their incapacities had been recognized early in life. Concomitantly, the parents seemed to be less consistent in demanding compliance from the schizophrenic child while expecting more responsible behavior from the siblings. When the ratings of the behavior of these parents were compared with data obtained by Bandura and Walters (1959) from parents of normal adolescent boys, it appeared that the families in the Sloat sample of preadolescent children were less open in expressing affection, less clear in spelling out their expectations to their children, less consistent, and more punitive in their dealing with unacceptable behavior. As far as the interviews could assess, these parents did not treat their schizo-phrenic child differently from his siblings, and some of the suggestive differences appeared to have been the consequences of the schizo-phrenic child's atypical state. In the absence of norms on parents of preadolescent children it is difficult to evaluate the reported differences between the parents in this sample and the parents of adolescents. If the parents in the Sloat study were indeed different, it would still be impossible to say whether this difference is related to their reaction to having a schizophrenic child and so Sloat's conclusion that they may provide a "pathological" environment for all their children, with the schizophrenic child being more affected, does not seem to rest on very firm foundation. Even if valid, the conclusion would still leave unanswered the question why the schizophrenic child would be more affected by the parents' deviant child-rearing behavior. Sloat suggested that it is either because the parents focus more on him or because predispositional factors make him more susceptible—a causal question that no correlational study can answer.

A comparison capable of throwing some light on the question whether parents' behavior undergoes changes in consequence of having an impaired child or whether the child's disorder is likely to have resulted from deviant parental behavior, calls—in the absence of controlled longitudinal studies—for a group of children whose condition is clearly congenital and thus not caused by influences in the social environment. *Cerebral palsy* is one such condition, for while the behavior of the child with this disorder will come to be molded by his experience, his physical condition antedates social interactions. If the experience of having an impaired child affects the mother's behavior, there should be no differences in the behavior of mothers of schizophrenic children and mothers of cerebral palsied children. On the other hand, if the mother's behavior somehow "causes" her child to become schizophrenic, the behavior of mothers of schizophrenic children should differ markedly from the behavior of mothers of other children. Klebanoff (1959) conducted a study relevant to this issue in that he compared maternal attitudes toward child rearing using mothers of schizophrenic children, of retarded and brain-injured children, and of healthy, normal children. He reported that the mothers of the schizophrenic children showed *fewer* "pathological" attitudes than the mothers of the brain-damaged and retarded children. Further, the mothers of the impaired children (including the schizophrenic) expressed more pathological attitudes than the mothers of the normal children, suggesting that deviant parental behavior may indeed be the reaction to and not the cause of deviant child behavior.

The results of a study conducted by Connerly (1967) also indicate that deviant parental behavior can easily be the result and not the cause of deviant child behavior. He compared parents of brain-injured children with parents of normal children, using instruments designed to elicit statements about child-rearing practices, personality characteristics, and anxiety level. The data led him to conclude that there were differences along these dimensions between his 30 parents of organically impaired children and the control group of parents of normal children. The parents of the normal children seemed less domineering and possessive and more relaxed with their child. The mothers seemed more secure in their concept of parenthood and less anxious about child-rearing than were the mothers of the brain-injured. In general, the home of the brain-injured child was described as less relaxed, as having more areas of conflict between father and mother, and having parents who expressed more omnipotent control over the child than was true in the case of the home of the normal child. Since brain injury, unlike the behavioral characteristics of the schizophrenic child, is difficult to construe as the result of parental attitudes, Connerly's data would suggest that the presence of a deviant child in the home can have a measurable effect on the parents' behavior.

A study by Shodell (1967) lends further support to this speculation. Her comparison was between mothers of cerebral palsied children, mothers of verbal schizophrenic children, and mothers of nonverbal schizophrenic children. There were 20 mothers in each group; they were matched for age, education, and family income; and the children—between the ages of five and twelve—were living at home and attended special day centers. Contrary to her hypothesis, Shodell did not find the mothers of the schizophrenic children to be "more immature and pathological" than the mothers of the cerebral palsied children, but the mothers of the schizophrenic did have higher anxiety scores on the MMPI measure. Anxiety scores also differentiated between the mothers of the nonverbal and the verbal schizophrenic children, but this finding was the reverse of what had been predicted, for the mothers of the verbal were less able to cope with their anxiety in a constructive fashion. These results led Shodell to draw a conclusion that posits an interaction effect whereby "some peculiarity in the infant behavior of the schizophrenic child may have provoked [the mother's] basic anxiety and affected her modes of controlling this anxiety." She further suggested that while the verbal and nonverbal schizophrenic children may be born with the same "basic endowments," the different ways in which their mothers dealt with their own reactive anxiety may have resulted in the differential speech development; the mothers of the nonverbal possibly having understimulated their children, while the mothers of the verbal schizophrenics possibly having become oversolicitous.

Nothing in available research lends support to the notion that psychotic or schizophrenic children are basically normal children who "were made psychotic" by some peculiarity in the behavior of their "schizophrenogenic" mother. The most conservative conclusion one can draw is that that diverse group of children—variously called *atypical, schizophrenic,* or *psychotic*—includes a large number whose profoundly disturbed behavior so upsets the equilibrium of their family interaction that their parents, and particularly their mothers, display disturbances in their own behavior. This clearly leaves the etiology of the child's problem an open question.

Research on Child Characteristics

Studies devoted to parental behavior were usually guided by the investigator's desire to test the hypothesis of material contribution to the development of psychotic children. Studies devoted to the characteristics of the psychotic child are frequently more exploratory in nature, seeking to establish how children in this group respond to various sensory, cognitive, or motor tasks.

A number of investigators who evaluated psychotic children have reported finding perceptual deficits and distortions. Thus, Hermelin and O'Conner (1967), having matched normal and psychotic children for mental age and having compared their performance on position and length discrimination problems, report that the psychotic have difficulties with such discriminations. Their results were similar to those of Berkowitz (1961) and Goldfarb (1961) who reported difficulties in directionality, 2-point threshold, figure-ground discrimination, and finger localization.

The impaired performance on tasks requiring responses to sensory stimuli can be interpreted as due to deficient sensory functions, limited integrative capacity, or impaired response facility. At the present time, it is impossible to conclude anything other than that the performance of children classified as psychotic differs from the performance of children considered normal. Whether one basic defect, such as impaired attention, underlies all of the performance deficits or whether the variety of children classified as psychotic or schizophrenic have a variety of deficits is a question only further research can resolve.

Clinical observers often report that children with psychotic disorders frequently explore objects by touch, smell, or taste, in seeming preference to visual examination. This apparent preference for the use of tactual and chemoreceptors was the basis of a study conducted by Schopler (1966) in which he compared visual and tactual receptor preferences of schizophrenic, normal, and retarded children. The 30 schizophrenic children ranged in age from 5 years, 6 months to 9 years, 5 months. A group of 15 mentally subnormal children of similar mental age and a group of 90 normal children of similar chronological age were used to obtain comparison data. In 4 standardized situations, each child was given the choice of playing with a primarily visual or a primarily tactual toy. In one situation, for example, the choice was between pushing a button that would activate a slide projector showing colored pictures or pressing a lever that produced moderate hand vibration. In another situation, the child had the choice between watching toy animals which were individually exposed by means of a rotating disk or tactually exploring similar animals enclosed in separate, screened compartments. Schopler reports that the normal children spent more time with the visual than with the tactual tasks and that the length of time spent on the visual tasks increased with age. The retarded children also showed a preference for the visual over the tactual; but for the schizophrenic children, this relationship did not appear, for they spent slightly more time at the tactual than at the visual tasks. Comparisons between the normal and the schizophrenic children showed the latter to have displayed less visual preference than same-aged normal children, although the schizophrenic did not spend more absolute time on tactual exploration than did the normal controls. The difference between the 2 groups is largely the result of the greater absolute amount of time the normal children were willing to spend on the various tasks, and of this time, they devoted more to the visual activities. Thus, the mean time spent on tactual stimuli was about $6\frac{1}{2}$ minutes (6.6) for the schizophrenic and a little over 6 minutes (6.2) for same-aged normal children. The mean time spent on visual stimuli, on the other hand, showed 6.2 minutes for the schizophrenic but 10.3 minutes for the normal comparison group of the same age.

Schopler (1966) concluded from his findings that "schizophrenic children will express less visual preference than normal children of the same age" (p. 113). A conclusion with somewhat better foundation in the data would seem to be that the normal children spent more time with the experimental tasks, and of that time, they spent more with the primarily visual than with the primarily tactual stimuli. The schizophrenic children spent less total time on the tasks than did the normal children, and the difference in total time represents the time the normal children spent with the visual stimuli. It seems tenuous to conclude that this is due to "less visual preference" on the part of the schizophrenic children. In the absence of significant differences between schizophrenics and normals on the tactual measures, the results may be as easily due to the characteristics of the stimulus material used in this study as to differences in receptor preference.

The comparatively limited amount of time a child with a psychotic disorder is willing to spend on tasks of interest to an experimenter—as opposed to the inordinate length of time they often spend on self-selected, repetitive, stereotyped activity—is frequently attributed to short attention span. Rutter and Lockyer (1967) for example, in comparing 63 children with infantile psychosis (probably including cases of early infantile autism) with a group of nonpsychotic, matched controls, list short attention span as one of the characteristics of their patients, but their list also includes stereotyped, repetitive mannerisms and nondistractibility. It would seem important to explore the dimension of stimulus characteristics before using the responses of psychotic children as a basis of drawing inferences about their preferences or ability to attend. Few investigators have addressed themselves to the question of the kinds of stimuli to which psychotic children do and do not respond. Work by Hermelin and O'Conner (1965, 1967) has some bearing on this, although their interest was primarily in discrimination learning. In one study (Hermelin & O'Conner, 1965) they compared speaking and nonspeaking psychotic children with normal controls of matched mental age on a series of visual discrimination tasks. They found that tasks that could be solved on the basis of kinesthetic, brightness, or size cues did not differentiate between the groups, while those tasks which required the discrimination of shape or direction presented difficulties for the psychotic subjects. In a later study (Hermelin & O'Conner, 1967) these investigators explored the dimensions of position and length in relation to the discrimination learning of 32 psychotic children and an equal number of normal controls of matched mental age. All subjects learned to discriminate position more readily than length, with the normal children superior to the psychotic children in the tasks requiring the discrimination of position.

When one wishes to investigate children's performance on tasks where verbal mediation may facilitate solution, as is the case in discrimination learning, matching groups on language development may be more relevant than matching them on the more general criterion of mental age. This emerged from a study conducted by Heller (1966) who investigated conceptual sorting of schizophrenic children. He initially matched 27 schizophrenic and 27 elementary school children by age, sex, intelligence and socioeconomic status. The minimal measured IQ score was 78. These subjects were given an object-sorting test that requires the classification of objects and the verbalization of the principle used in the sorting. The test was scored in terms of the adequacy of the sorting and of the verbalizations. The schizophrenic subjects were found to give a significantly greater number of idiosyncratic verbalizations, but only the older schizophrenic children displayed less adequate sorting than their normal controls. These differences, however, became negligible when the two groups were equated for language development. This seems to suggest that such differences as had been found between the two groups were largely a function of the language impairment of the schizophrenic children. Heller concluded that the inadequate language development of schizophrenic children results in an inability to focus on relevant aspects of the environment, leading to irrelevant, idiosyncratic, maladaptive, and bizarre associations and responses. Unable to reduce stimulus complexity through verbal labeling, the schizophrenic child would have difficulty in dealing with the events around him and to orient himself in relation to his environment.

The importance of language in the development and course of children's psychotic disorders is also reflected in the finding of Rutter, Greenfeld, and Lockyer (1967) that psychotic children who fail to develop useful language by age five are far less likely to show later improvement than those whose language development is less impaired. This is, of course, another way of saying that the more severe the disorder, the greater the language impairment and the less favorable the prognosis. From this one might also conclude that the earlier one intervenes and gives the child systematic language training and other treatment aimed at enhancing the socialization process, the more likely one will be to promote adaptive development.

Critique

Studies such as those just reviewed throw some light on the differences in performance between normal children and a heterogeneous group of profoundly disturbed children. Differences do seem to exist, but beyond that self-evident statement, there is little one can offer by way of an integrating conclusion. Aside from the problem of definition which, until solved, continues to lead different investigators to study different children while calling them by the same catchall labels, there is the handicap of doing research without a guiding theory that might permit one to generate testable hypotheses. With few exceptions (Schopler, 1965), studies of the sensory and re-sponse capacities of psychotic children seem to be approached in the exploratory spirit of "I-wonder-what-would-happen-if." This is a reflection of the rudimentary state of knowledge in which we find ourselves in this field, for such an approach is typical of a very early period in scientific endeavor. In addition to this lack of a theory, there are methodological issues which must be solved before much progress can be expected.

One methodological problem that faces investigators interested in the learning capacity of psychotic children is the kind of control group which should be used in order to isolate the "psychotic" variable. Children with psychotic disorders are observed to have difficulty learning to discriminate objects by their shape, for example. It is also known, however, that these children obtain very low mental-age scores on tests of intelligence. If one now desired to demonstrate that shape discrimination is more difficult for psychotic than for normal children, what kind of "normal" children should one use for comparison? This question arises because investigators wish to study whether the difficulty with shape discrimination is "due to" the psychotic condition or "caused by" the psychotic child's low mental age. Hermelin and O'Conner (1967) attempted to solve this issue by matching for mental age. Since the measurable mental age of the psychotic subjects was less than half their chronological age, this meant that they had to select very young, normal children for their control group. As a result, the mean chronological age of the normal children was 4 years, 4 months, while the mean chronological age of their patient group was 11 years. This discrepancy in chrono-logical age introduces factors into the study that may grossly distort the results. For example, the nature of the game, toy, or reward or the size of a manipulandum appropriate for an eleven-year-old will be inappropriate for a four-year-old and vice versa, regardless of psychotic condition or intelligence level. Such differences as may be found between these groups may thus be due to factors other than or in addition to the psychotic condition of the patient group.

The study by Schopler (1966), discussed above, used two control groups—one matched for mental age, the other matched for chronological age. Since the differences in time spent on the visual, as opposed to the tactual, tasks was found to hold regardless of the mental age of the control group, Schopler concluded that it was not a function of the low intelligence level of his psychotic children, implying that it was therefore a function of the fact that they were psychotic or schizophrenic. While two control groups permit one to make statements about the effect of the intelligence variable, they still do not provide a basis for speculations about the effect of the psychotic condition on, say, shape discrimination. This is the case because mental age is not a measure that is independent of the psychotic condition. Mental age is no more than a score a child achieves on an intelligence test. When a child with a psychotic disorder is tested, his test performance is going to be influenced by his disorder, and his score is going to reflect his condition. If this child is then also tested on a shape-discrimination task and he is found to have difficulty with this, it is meaningless to ask whether his difficulty is the result of his "low intelligence" or due to his psychotic condition. The most parsimonious statement one can make is that the poor performance on the test of intelligence (which calls for shape discriminations, among other things) and his poor performance on an experimental task requiring shape discrimination are some of the many forms of maladaptive behavior that, together, have come to be called *psychosis* or *schizophrenia*.

The various behaviors making up the vague cluster labeled *psychotic disorders* are described in the nine characteristics cited at the beginning of this chapter. Ultimately, studies, such as those by Schopler (1966) and Hermelin and O'Conner (1967), do no more than show that some of these characteristics are indeed intercorrelated and that children who are called *normal* do not show these characteristics. What makes some children manifest these characteristics and so come to be called *psychotic* or *schizophrenic*—the "cause" of the condition—remains to be discovered.

Follow-up Studies

The work of Rutter and Lockyer (1967) and of Rutter, Greenfeld, and Lockyer (1967) represents the most ambitious attempt thus far to provide information on the development of children with psychotic disorders. These reports provide a 5-to 15-year follow-up of children who had been designated as cases of "infantile psychosis." These children had been hospitalized between 1950 and 1958, and the follow-up was conducted in 1963 and 1964. Because the issue of nomenclature was even more confused in the 1950s than it is now, the cases included children with a variety of psychotic disorders, including early infantile autism. "Most" had shown psychotic development in early infancy, and their principal characteristics were distorted relationship with people, marked retardation of language, echolalia and pronominal reversal, stereotyped, repetitive mannerisms, a lack of responsiveness to auditory stimuli, and a tendency to self-injurious behavior. Rutter and his colleagues (1967) compared the later status of 63 such children with that of a matched, nonpsychotic control group of children who, at one time, had been patients at the same psychiatric hospital during that 8-year period. The psychotic children had a mean age of 5 years, 11 months at the time of the original hospitalization. The average intelligence quotient of the 53 who could be tested had been 62.5. None had shown "unequivocal" signs of central nervous system abnormality during the physical examination at time of admission. The male/female ratio was 4.25 to 1, reflecting the repeatedly reported disproportionate representation of boys among severely disturbed children. When the mean age of the psychotic children was 15 years, 7 months, they were reexamined with Rutter and his colleagues personally conducting the examination in all but 2 instances. The most noteworthy result of the study is that follow-up revealed a high incidence of brain damage among the psychotic. Of the 63 children who, on original examination, had shown no clear-cut abnormality, only 29 showed no evidence of brain damage when they were reexamined. The presence of brain damage was considered a "strong likelihood" in 12 cases, 10 of whom had developed epileptic seizures. In 6 cases brain damage was deemed "probable," and in another 16 cases the presence of such impairment was classified as "possible." This change in diagnostic picture may, of course, be an artifact of more sophisticated examination, but the finding of high incidence of brain damage among psychotic children is in line with data presented by Eaton and Menolascino (1967) on the basis of their 5-year follow-up of 32 psychotic children. Eaton and Menolascino view brain-damaged children as unusually reactive to stress and suggest that some psychotic reactions of childhood are secondary to central nervous system impairment.

The primary interest of the research by Rutter and his associates (1967) was to ascertain the social adjustment of their 2 groups of children. For this purpose they assigned Social Adjustment Ratings on a 4-point scale. These ratings are shown in Table 2. As can be seen from this table, the psychotic group had attained a far worse

Table 2

Social Adjustment Ratings at Follow-up*

Rating	Percent Psychotic	Percent Non-psychotic
Normal/Good	14	33
Fair	25	31
Poor	13	11
Very Poor	48	25

*After Rutter, Greenfeld, and Lockyer, 1967, p. 1184.

level of adjustment than the comparison group of nonpsychotic psychiatric patients. Only 1 case in the psychotic group was reported to have fully normal peer relations, and only 7 were able to relate to adults in a fully normal manner. The social-adjustment ratings which may be subjectively biased receive more objective support from the data on the settings in which the subjects were located at the time of follow-up (Table 3). All but 5 (8 percent) of the psychotic group were in some specialized, sheltered, or institutional setting. In the comparison group 21 individuals (34 percent) were either employed or attending ordinary school. When those over age 16 are separately scrutinized, one finds that only 2 (5 percent) of the psychotic but 12 (33 percent) of the nonpsychotic expatients are listed as employed. A large proportion of both groups (44 percent of the psychotic and 36 percent of the nonpsychotic) were found on follow-up

Table 3

Status at Follow-up*

Status	All Subjects		Subjects over Age 16	
	Psychotic	Control	Psychotic	Control
Employed	2	14	2	12
Regular school	3	7	1	...
Special school	11	6	1	3
Living in village trust	3	...	3	...
Training center	7	10	4	6
At home, not working	9	2	7	1
Institutionalized	28	22	20	14
Total	63	61	38	36

*After Rutter, Greenfeld, and Lockyer, 1967, p. 1184.

to be institutionalized, primarily in institutions for the mentally retarded. This reflects both the shortage of appropriate facilities for
severely disturbed children and youth and the low reliability of
nomenclature and resulting arbitrary dispositions in this field. The
bimodal distribution for the comparison group (34 percent in
regular school or employment and 36 percent in institutions) reflects the heterogeneous nature of this group, some of whom had
originally come into psychiatric care because of severe acting out
and delinquency, while others had been hospitalized because of
questionable retardation or brain damage.

Rutter, Greenfeld, and Lockyer (1967) point out that their
results are similar to those of other investigators, such as Eisenberg
(1956), who conducted follow-up studies on severely disturbed,
autistic children and found some 50 percent to have been institutionalized by adolescence, again usually in institutions for the mentally retarded. Only from between 5 and 17 percent of these children

were rated as "well adjusted," and even those whose autistic withdrawal was attenuated continued to show a lack of perceptiveness for the nuances of social behavior, such as interpersonal tact.

The low rate of positive outcomes in cases of childhood psychosis is, of course, closely related to the inadequacy, inefficiency, and sheer lack of available treatment resources. The children in the study by Rutter et al. had been exposed to an extremely heterogeneous range of "treatments," including prolonged, daily psychoanalytic therapy, routine institutional care, medications of various kinds, and—in one instance—a leucotomy (accounting for one case of brain damage!). Treatment form seemed unrelated to outcome, with one notable exception: the amount of schooling. This, together with initial intelligence level, the presence or absence of speech by age five, and the overall severity of the disorder, was a main variable that was clearly related to outcome. All children in the "good" outcome category (Table 2) had attended school for at least 2 years. This was true of only 63 percent of the "fair," 38 percent of the "poor," and 20 percent of the "very poor" outcome groups. The ability to attend school was only partly related to original intelligence level as indicated by the fact that intelligence level did not differentiate between the "good" and "fair" groups who differed significantly on the school attendance variable. It would thus seem incorrect to attribute the positive relationship between school attendance and outcome to the fact that the less severely disturbed who were able to attend school had a higher probability of receiving a good adjustment rating on follow-up. Schooling appeared to contribute to positive outcome in its own right, somewhat independent of the initial level of the disturbance. As Rutter and his colleagues point out, "schooling probably did have some effect on the child's social adjustment in adolescence and early life" (1967, p. 1195). In the group these investigators had studied, fewer than 50 percent of the psychotic children had as much as 2 years of regular school attendance while 33 percent had never been exposed to school, 10 percent had gone to school for less than 6 months, and 6 percent had received some schooling only during their original, short hospitalization. Greater efforts at providing these children appropriate, individualized, systematic educational opportunities might well increase their chances for greatly improved functioning, justifying Rutter, Greenfeld, and Lockyer's "limited optimism" that with better facilities, better results might be obtained.

RECAPITULATION

There is little agreement regarding the terminology to describe a child whose withdrawn behavior is so pervasive that it distorts and disrupts his relationship with the world around him. The most commonly used term for children whose disorders have psychotic dimensions is childhood schizophrenia, but, like all other arbitrary labels, this one raises more questions than it answers. Regarding etiology, the best available data suggest that the excessive avoidance responses of these children have their basis in an interaction between neurophysiological and environmental factors. There is little to substantiate the hypothesis that either or both parents "cause" the child's problem. On the contrary, it may well be that the presence of a profoundly disturbed child in the home has a disrupting effect on family equilibrium and parental behavior. Most treatments presently in use show singularly poor results, and the only approach permitting a "limited optimism" seems to take the form of systematic, individualized educational efforts. Such efforts are closely related to the treatment approaches discussed in the following chapters, approaches which view treatment primarily as a matter of learning, unlearning, and relearning.

PART IV

THE TREATMENT OF PSYCHOLOGICAL DISORDERS

12

BEHAVIOR THERAPY: PREMISES AND PRINCIPLES

The study of the psychological disorders of children would be an idle intellectual exercise were it not to result in action designed to help children who have such disorders. In keeping with the orientation that guided the previous chapters, this discussion of treatment will focus on the behavioral approaches currently in use, approaches which are generally known as *behavior therapy.*

The modern origins of behavior therapy with children can be traced to 1924, the year Mary Cover Jones published the case of Peter whose generalized fear of furry objects she had treated by the application of the principles of respondent conditioning. A few years later, Krasnogorski (1925), Ivanov-Smolenski (1927), and Gesell (1938) pointed to the relevance of Pavlovian conditioning to the treatment of psychological disorders. But it seems that the time was not ripe for this obvious suggestion, for although Mowrer and Mowrer (1938) described the treatment of bed-wetting by conditioning techniques in the intervening years, it was not until Skinner (1953), Eysenck (1957), Wolpe (1958), and Bandura (1961) pointed out that laboratory-derived and laboratory-tested methods could be applied to the modification of psychological disorders that behavior therapy became more widely used.

While the prototype of this form of treatment had been a three-year-old boy (Jones, 1924a), early application of behavior therapy was almost entirely limited to adults, and 20 years after Jones had treated little Peter, only occasional reports dealing with the treatment of children had appeared in the literature (Ross, 1964a). While some publications in South Africa (Lazarus, 1959) and Great Britain (Jones, 1960) dealt with child cases, it was not until approaches based on the principles of operant conditioning were used in work with institutionalized children (Ferster & DeMyer, 1962) that behavior therapy became more widely applied in the treatment of children. By the time Gelfand and Hartman prepared a review published in 1968, they were able to cite some seventy references.

THE PREMISES OF THE BEHAVIOR THERAPIST

Behavior therapy is an approach to the alleviation of psychological problems which rests on the premise that these problems represent learned maladaptive behavior or a failure to have learned adaptive behavior. The focus is on behavior as it can be observed in the here-and-now, and the aim of the behavior therapist is to change that behavior in the adaptive direction. His premise leads the behavior therapist to seek behavior change through the application of various psychological principles that derive from research in the laboratory where learning has long been the object of systematic study. In the application of these principles various methods may come to be used, and behavior therapy cannot be viewed as synonymous with any one method or technique.

As was pointed out in Chapter 1, behavior that is observed at any point in time represents the end point of the interaction of four variables: genetic-constitutional endowment, past learning, the individual's current physiological state, and his current environmental conditions. Of these four, only two are subject to manipulation by a therapist wishing to induce behavior change; these are the current environmental conditions and the individual's physiological state. Since the physiological state is, in turn, changeable only by changing environmental conditions, the focus of behavior therapy falls on the environment in which the individual currently lives. The emphasis on the current situation is one of the defining characteristics of behavior therapy. Whether the problem be one of excess or of deficient behavior, the behavior therapist intensively studies what is going on in the here-and-now and makes his remedial plans on the basis of information thus obtained. While the learning orientation logically implies the recognition of the fact that past events contributed to the development of present difficulties, the behavior therapist considers a detailed knowledge of the person's history unessential for planning or conducting therapy.

If it were possible to obtain a factual account of the conditions under which maladaptive behavior was acquired together with an accurate statement of the child's reinforcement history, such knowledge might aid a therapist in deciding on the most suitable approach to treatment. Unfortunately, information of this kind is not available. Several studies (e.g., Wenar, 1961 ; Robbins, 1963) have shown that the developmental "histories" obtained from mothers are neither reliable nor valid, and for this reason it would seem that a therapist's efforts can be put to better advantage than to try and gather such material.

The focus of behavior therapy is on current behavior and its current circumstances, and this focus guides the work of the behavior therapist from the beginning of his contact with his client. As Kanfer and Phillips (1966) have pointed out, a behavioral approach must entail more than the application of learning principles to treatment as such; the behavioral approach must be reflected in all aspects of the clinical contact. This means that the expectations with which parents and child enter the contact must be relevant to the orientation on which the helping process is to be based. Since the general public has a stereotyped notion of the nature of psychotherapy that is based on traditional approaches, this frequently means that the set with which a family comes for help must be modified in the initial contacts. Beyond this, however, the assessment phase of the contact must be guided by the behavioral orientation.

When a task at hand is to treat an individual child, the focus of assessment is not "How did he get this way?" but "What must be done to help him acquire more adaptive behavior?" Assessment covers a wide range of factors that *currently* play a role in the child's life, including his physical state, his constitutional capacity, his intellectual ability, and his sociofamilial environment. There are four questions to which answers must be found:

1. What is the child's current response repertoire, including the maladaptive responses that brought him to the clinician?

2. What is the intensity, rate, strength, or frequency of the maladaptive responses?

3. Under what circumstances (antecedents and consequences) are the maladaptive responses emitted?

4. What environmental conditions in the child's life lend themselves to therapeutic manipulation?

Once the answers to these questions are ascertained through careful interview and observation, the next question becomes "What is to be the treatment goal and how can it best be reached?"

At the present time, these questions must be answered through interview and observation of behavior because the development of assessment techniques relevant to behavior therapy has lagged behind the development of the treatment procedures themselves. As Goodkin (1967) pointed out, there is a dearth of methods designed to select appropriate target behaviors, appropriate treatment methods, and suitable reinforcers. Since the reactions of the social environment are an important consequence of behavior which often has reinforcing capacity, adequate assessment for behavior therapy should include data on the kind of reactions a child elicits from others and the kind of behaviors which elicit these reactions. This point was stressed by Patterson, Jones, Whittier, and Wright (1965) who suggest that if it were possible to select for modification that response which is most likely to effect a change in the reactions of others and particularly of the peer group, treatment might be enhanced through the generalization of its effects. Rather than devising a treatment procedure to modify each of a child's problematic behaviors singly and separately, the therapist could maximize his effectiveness by selecting for treatment that behavior on which other problem behaviors depend. An example of this was presented in the discussion of enuresis (Chapter 8) where it has been found that treatment often results in improvements in such untreated areas as peer relations, school achievement, and interactions within the family.

THEORETICAL BACKGROUND

The behavior therapist seeks to apply known psychological principles in the treatment of behavior disorders. In the case of deficient behavior the therapeutic task is to establish missing responses; in the case of excess behavior, the child must learn to modify these responses so as to make his behavior more adaptive to the demands of his environment. In either case, treatment involves learning, unlearning, and relearning. The principles of learning which behavior therapists bring to bear on the analysis and modification of behavior disorders can be discussed under three headings—respondent conditioning, operant conditioning, and observational learning—although the three may well represent different aspects of the same basic process, and they assuredly interact whenever human learning takes place in a natural environment.

Respondent Conditioning

At times called *Pavlovian* or *classical conditioning*, this kind of learning involves the modification of a response that the organism is innately capable of making by substituting a conditioned stimulus for the natural or unconditioned stimulus. A well-known example is the case of little Albert (Watson & Raynor, 1920) who was conditioned to make a fear response to the stimulus of a white rat by having the rat repeatedly paired with a loud noise—a stimulus that elicits fear, apparently innately. Prior to this conditioning, the rat had been an object of curiosity to the child who was thus shown to have learned to fear the animal. It is a distinctive aspect of respondent conditioning that an innate response is *elicited* by a stimulus which *precedes* it and that the organism is *passively responding* to potent environmental events or external stimuli. The responses in question usually involve the autonomic nervous system, and respondent conditioning is probably always involved when emotional responses come to be attached to previously neutral stimuli.

A number of phenomena that have been intensively studied in the psychological laboratory are of particular relevance to the behavior therapist. These are stimulus generalization, extinction, conditioned inhibition, and differential inhibition. Wolpe (1958) and others, who treat maladaptive emotional reactions by what they variously call counterconditioning or reciprocal inhibition, produce a decrement of a conditioned response by eliciting an incompatible response to the same conditioned stimulus.

Operant Conditioning

In respondent conditioning, the environment elicits a response from a primarily passive organism. The situation is essentially reversed in the case of operant conditioning. Here the organism actively emits a response to which the environment reacts; in other words, the response is instrumental in bringing about an environmental event. The importance of this sequence lies in the fact that it is the *consequence* of the response that serves to change the probability of that response's recurrence under similar conditions at a later time. The conditions (stimuli) under which the organism has encountered certain consequences to his response will come to control this response in the sense that the response will occur with greater probability when these conditions pertain than when they do not, but the conditions do not elicit the response, as does the conditioned stimulus in the case of respondent conditioning. Operant behavior is a function of its consequences, and when such behavior is to be modified, the contingencies under which these consequences occur must be changed (Skinner, 1938).

In technical terminology the sequence of operant conditioning is the presence of a discriminative stimulus, the emission of an operant response, and the presentation of a reinforcing stimulus which is usually followed by a consummatory response. The discriminative stimulus thus represents a signal that indicates the likelihood of the appearance of the reinforcing stimulus once the response has been emitted. As a signal, it may or may not have an effect on the organism, depending on his then current state which is a function of such "setting events" as deprivation or satiation for the particular reinforcer.

Since the operant response cannot be reinforced until it has been emitted, the response must be one that is already in the organism's repertoire. Where this is not the case, someone in the environment—parent, teacher, or therapist—must select a similar, already established response and, by selectively reinforcing successive approximations of the desired response, "shape" the necessary behavior.

As in respondent conditioning, the stimulus in operant conditioning exhibits the phenomenon of stimulus generalization. That is, not only the original discriminative stimulus but also the range of similar stimuli come to be capable of controlling the response. The more similar these stimuli are to the original, the greater will be the probability that the learned response will occur. On the other hand, a learned response that is repeatedly emitted in the absence of reinforcing consequences will gradually occur with decreasing probability, a process that is labeled *extinction* in both operant and respondent conditioning.

Inasmuch as the operant response is a function of its consequences, an examination of possible consequences is essential if one is to attempt the modification of a response. Consequences can fall in one of three classes: positive, negative, or neutral. Positive consequences will strengthen the response in the sense that they will increase the likelihood of its recurrence under similar circumstances; negative consequences will reduce the likelihood of the response, i.e., they will weaken it; while neutral consequences, being those that have no reinforcing effect, will result in extinction. There are two conditions that can represent positive consequences and two that can represent negative consequences. The presentation of a satisfying stimulation (reward) or the termination or avoidance of noxious stimulation (negative reinforcement) both represent positive consequences, while the presentation of noxious stimulation (punishment) or the removal of satisfying stimulation (time-out from positive reinforcement) both represent negative consequences.

It will be apparent that when either positive or negative stimulation is to be withdrawn, the relevant stimulation must already be present. Similarly, positive reinforcement depends for its effectiveness on the setting condition of deprivation. This makes the delivery of noxious stimulation the only manipulation that can be presented without preparation and regardless of the condition of the organism; yet despite its ready availability, punishment is complex both in its effect and in its current theoretical status in learning research.

Among the effects of punishment appears to be a physiological arousal state that can become conditioned to the stimuli present when punishment is delivered. While these stimuli may be relevant to the particular behavior being punished so that this behavior will come to be avoided or suppressed by incompatible responses, the stimuli may also be relevant to the person delivering the noxious stimulation so that this person will come to elicit fear and hence avoidance or escape responses.

In addition to these emotional and interpersonal aspects of punishment, there is the consideration that it does not actually eliminate the punished behavior but that it simply leads to a suppression of the behavior because of the arousal of incompatible emotional responses and their consequences. Punished behavior will only remain suppressed as long as conditional aversive stimuli are present; once these are absent, the punished behavior will reappear, particularly where it carries its own natural reinforcer, as in the case of taking cookies out of the cooky jar. For this reason, it is important that punishment, when used in treatment or child rearing, be paired with positive reinforcement of desirable responses that are incompatible with the responses to be weakened.

A phenomenon which permits a wide range of stimuli to serve as reinforcers is that variously called *conditioned, secondary,* or *acquired reinforcement.* A previously neutral event that repeatedly precedes a reinforcing stimulus takes on reinforcing properties in its own right. This makes it possible to reinforce a child's responses not only with such primary reinforcers as food but also by such secondary reinforcers as approval, praise, tokens, or grades on report cards. Premack (1959) has pointed out that a response with high probability of occurrence can be used to reinforce a response of lower probability. In the case of children this means that play can be used to reinforce work, shouting can reinforce being quiet, etc. The principle of secondary reinforcement also holds in the case of punishment. Thus, when verbal reprimands, frowns, or threats have been paired with the administration of more direct, physical punishment or the removal of positive stimulation, the more symbolic, social stimuli can acquire punishing properties in their own right.

Observational Learning

When a response is not in an individual's repertoire, the principle of operant conditioning demands that the desired response must be "shaped" by reinforcing successive approximations. Bandura (1969) has pointed out that the painstaking process of successive approximations is so inefficient that it lacks survival value in natural settings and is thus likely to work best under contrived laboratory conditions. Bandura has been instrumental in calling attention to a learning process that seems to play a major role in socialization, the process of observational learning.

When an observer watches a model engage in a given behavior, three effects can be observed. The observer may acquire new response patterns, previously not in his behavior repertoire; the consequences of the modeled action to the performer may strengthen or weaken the observer's inhibitory responses; and the observer's previously learned behavior in the same general class as that displayed by the model may be facilitated. Bandura (1969) stresses that the *acquisition* of the response does not require reinforcement of the observer at the time of observing but that the *performance* of the vicariously learned response may depend on reinforcement contingencies. At the same time, observational learning requires more than exposing an individual to modeling stimuli, and the absence of appropriate matching responses following such exposure may result from a variety of factors such as the observer's failure to have attended to the relevant stimuli, his failure to retain what he has learned, a motor deficit that makes it impossible for him to perform the response or unfavorable conditions of reinforcement.

Research conducted by Bandura (see Bandura, 1969 for an authoritative summary) demonstrates convincingly that observational learning is enhanced when the model's behavior receives positive reinforcement, when the model holds higher status than the observer, and when the model is in a power position with regard to the observer. Since not only motor responses but also cognitive attitudinal and emotional responses can be acquired through observational learning, its role in socialization would seem to be immense and its contribution to therapy highly promising.

IMPLICATIONS FOR TREATMENT

As this cursory summary of theoretical principles and pragmatic statements suggests, a variety of approaches are available to the therapist wishing to modify the problematic behavior of a child. When the problem takes the form of a behavioral deficit, the responses missing from the child's repertoire must be established; while in the case of excess behavior, the responses in question can be modified, reduced, or eliminated and replaced by more adaptive behavior. Often, as in the case of the autistic child, some behavior (e.g., speech) must be established while other behavior (e.g., head banging) has to be reduced, but no matter how complex, the necessary modifications of behavior invariably entail learning.

The various approaches available to the behavior therapist can be used alone or in combination and the choice depends, in part, on the specific needs of the case and the conditions under which treatment can be carried out. In the most general sense, the respondent conditioning paradigm can be viewed as best suited for the treatment of problems in the vascular-visceral-autonomic realm (e.g., fears), while the operant approach lends itself best to problems involving skeletal-muscular-motor functions (e.g., hitting or speech). This distinction follows the logic of a 2-factor theory of learning (Mowrer, 1951; Rescorla & Solomon, 1967), but recent research (e.g., Katkin & Murray, 1968) has demonstrated that visceral responses can be modified through operant conditioning so that it is probably overly simplistic to assign autonomic responses to the respondent and voluntary responses to the operant conditioning realm. Furthermore, with the explication of observational learning by Bandura (1969) who has shown that emotional responses, motor skills, and complex social behavior can be learned vicariously, it has become apparent that behavior therapy is never purely respondent, purely operant, or purely observational. The therapist may wish to focus his activity on one or the other of these paradigms, but all three will undoubtedly enter into the situation, no matter what he does.

The therapist's choice of which paradigm to use as a focus will often be guided by the degree of cooperation he can expect from his child client. In respondent conditioning, where the therapist presents stimuli to the child, it would appear that the child is a passive recipient of therapy and that he merely reacts with elicited responses. Despite this apparent passivity of the child, it would be wrong to conclude that the therapist manipulates an unwilling or unwitting "victim," for unlike the animal in the classical conditioning experiment, the child is not in a restraining harness. He is quite able not to attend to the stimuli presented to him, not to remain in the room, or to emit responses that are incompatible with those the therapist is trying to elicit. These circumstances make respondent conditioning treatment best suited to situations where children are motivated for getting help with a problem they recognize as troubling them. Cooperation in treatment is essential, and since this is more likely to be found with less severely impaired and older children in non-residential clinic settings, it is there that this form of treatment is likely to be successful.

Where the operant conditioning paradigm guides the treatment approach, the child is a very active participant because he engages in an operation—does something to the environment. The therapist arranges the environment in such a way as to assure that the child's operant responses occur under particular conditions and are followed by planned consequences. This contingency management requires that the therapist have some control over the stimulus and reinforcement conditions that the child will encounter, and the level of possible control will largely determine the effectiveness with which treatment can be conducted. Inasmuch as a therapist's opportunity for such control is greatest in an institutional setting where, with the help of institutional personnel, he can influence the delivery of primary and secondary reinforcers, most reports of treatment using operant methods have come from such settings. In order to conduct this form of treatment in nonresidential settings, the therapist will need to obtain the close cooperation of the child's parents or teachers since these are in a better position to manage reinforcement contingencies than a therapist who has only occasional contact with the child.

In order to use observational learning as the principle focus of treatment, a therapist would need an appropriate and potent model or models and a child-client whom he can induce to observe these models engage in the behavior the child is expected to acquire and perform. This, again, requires cooperation on the part of the child-client and a setting, such as a normal nursery school, where other children model age-appropriate behavior. An institutional setting where other children tend to model inappropriate behavior is thus not the place to attempt treatment by vicarious learning. In fact, as Estes (1970) has suggested, one source of the behavioral deterioration found in children who are institutionalized for long periods of time, such as mental defectives, may be the presence of inappropriate peer models whose influence is countertherapeutic.

As stated previously, complex human learning, particularly in a social situation, entails operant, respondent, and observational aspects, and the same is true of the complex human learning called *therapy*. An example of the interrelationship of operant and respondent factors can be taken from the treatment of deficient control over eliminative functions.

By the time a child who has not learned age-appropriate toilet behavior comes to treatment, he is likely to have acquired, as a result of punishment experiences in connection with toilet training, at least some conditioned anxiety to stimuli associated with wetting or soiling. While treatment can be planned in terms of the operant paradigm, such that appropriate toilet behavior receives positive reinforcement (e.g., Neale, 1963), respondent factors will also play a role because each time an appropriate toilet response is made, anxiety that had become associated with soiling is being avoided. As frequency of soiling decreases, the anxiety associated with it will also decrease in frequency, and the training sequence must therefore be viewed as involving more than simple operant conditioning as Hundziak,

Maurer, and Watson (1965) have mistakenly suggested. This is especially the case where aversive stimuli and negative reinforcement are introduced in connection with the training procedure, as in the work by Giles and Wolf (1966) who also thought that their approach was purely operant.

It is unlikely that any complex learning can ever be said to be purely operant or purely respondent, and specific cases may indeed be best treated if the therapist explicitly plans a combination of operant and respondent approaches, as was the case in the work with a nine-year-old, school-phobic boy reported by Lazarus, Davison, and Polefka (1965). Assessment of this boy's problem revealed that his school-phobic behavior involved not only an intense fear of the school situation itself but also the fact that avoiding school was being maintained by attention and other secondary reinforcers delivered by parents, siblings, and therapists. It was therefore decided to treat the high level of anxiety by respondent (counterconditioning) techniques in the early phases of treatment and then to introduce operant strategies by making positive reinforcements contingent on school attendance. In order to assure treatment effectiveness, the different techniques had to be carefully chosen and properly timed with anxiety level at each stage of treatment carefully assessed.

Lazarus, Davison, and Polefka (1965) stress the risk involved in the inappropriate use of the operant model by pointing out that under conditions of high anxiety, premature exposure to the feared school situation would probably lead to heightened sensitivity and further escape and avoidance responses, which are reinforced by anxiety reduction. Conversely, treatment can also be impeded by the inappropriate use of the respondent model because attempts to induce relaxation and give reassurance may provide positive reinforcement, thus strengthening dependent, school-avoiding behavior.

The rudiments of the basic principles of behavior therapy are relatively easy to grasp, making it appear simple and easy to apply. This apparent simplicity should not lead anyone to believe that behavior therapy can be planned and directed by untrained or poorly trained individuals. The treatment is not without its risks. Mary Cover

Jones (1924b) recognized this long ago when she wrote regarding her pioneering work with Peter:

> This method obviously requires delicate handling. Two response systems are being dealt with: food leading to a positive re-action, and fear-object leading to a negative reaction. The desired conditioning should result in transforming the fear-object into a source of positive response (substitute stimulus). But a careless manipulator could readily produce the reverse result, attaching a fear reaction to the sight of food (p. 388).

13

TREATMENT
APPROACHES – I

This discussion of treatment approaches currently used in behavior therapy with children will be organized around the major aims of the intervention; that is, whether the therapeutic task is to increase or to decrease a target behavior. Depending on the nature of the problem, the therapist may need to increase desirable responses whose frequency is too low, or he may need to decrease the frequency of behaviors which are a problem because they occur in excess of the socially acceptable limits. This dichotomy into deficient and excess behavior is a handy device for organizing the material, but, as Gelfand and Hartman (1968) have pointed out, the multiple problems seen in clinical settings usually require a combination of approaches where the acceleration of the frequency of prosocial behaviors goes hand in hand with the elimination of problem behaviors. In fact, as has been pointed out repeatedly in earlier chapters, it is not sufficient to reduce the frequency of an excess behavior; the therapeutic task is not completed unless the child has learned adaptive responses which can take the place of the maladaptive, excess responses the therapist seeks to eliminate from his repertoire.

PROBLEMS OF DEFICIENT BEHAVIOR

At times it may seem difficult to decide whether a specific problem calls for acceleration or deceleration in response frequency because the direction of desired change often depends on how a problem is construed. In the case of bed-wetting, for example, one could say that the problem lies in deficient sphincter control or in excessive urination under improper conditions (in bed). It is only when one asks what the child will have to learn in order to overcome his problem that the decision of whether his difficulty is an excess or a deficit becomes clear. In the case of the example, the focus would be on establishing sphincter control, and the problem was thus classified as a behavior deficit for earlier presentation (Chapter 8). This logic also guides the following discussion.

Problems with Elimination

A common behavior deficit among children is lack of adequate sphincter control and the resulting incontinence of urine (enuresis) or feces (encopresis). The treatment of enuresis by the application of conditioning principles has been available for many years, having been described by Mowrer and Mowrer in 1938. In the basic bell-and-pad approach, the child sleeps on a pad that is wired in such a fashion that a single drop of urine will close a circuit and activate a bell or buzzer which continues to sound until it is manually turned off, either by the child or an attendant.

Werry (1966) reviewed twenty reports on the treatment of enuresis by conditioning techniques and concluded that it is generally effective. A comparative study by DeLeon and Mandell (1966) found conditioning techniques superior to traditional psychotherapeutic methods which are based on the assumption that bed-wetting is a symptom of an underlying, unconscious conflict. While the conditioning approach to the treatment of nocturnal enuresis has thus been found to work, the question of the mode in which it works has not yet been satisfactorily answered. Lovibond (1963) raised the issue whether this form of treatment represents an instance of classical conditioning, wherein the response of sphincter contraction is learned to the stimulus of bladder distension, or whether it should be viewed as avoidance learning in which case the contraction would represent the response that avoids the loud and sleep-disrupting noise. An experiment (Lovibond, 1964) designed to compare these alternative explanations favored the avoidance-conditioning formulation, but a more recent investigation by Turner, Young, and Rachman (1970) found no support for this hypothesis. This group of investigators compared the effectiveness of three signaling modes in order to ascertain whether louder, continuous, more unpleasant noises result in more rapid learning than an intermittent sound. Using a placebo and a wake-up control, they found the three conditioning methods equally effective with an initial success rate of 81.4 percent. On the other hand, they, like Lovibond (1963), noted a high relapse rate regardless of the conditioning method used.

The relapse rate in the treatment of enuresis may be viewed as a reflection of the fact that in this, as in similar cases of the treatment of behavior deficits, one is not merely establishing a response that was previously missing from the child's repertoire but that one is introducing into the repertoire a response that is antagonistic to one already established. An enuretic child is not simply one who lacks appropriate sphincter control; he is one who makes a micturition response to the stimulus of bladder distension. The therapeutic task must thus be viewed as establishing a complex series of behaviors that includes sustained sphincter contraction and micturition under appropriate stimulus conditions (toilet). One must thus strengthen an adaptive response pattern while simultaneously weakening its maladaptive reciprocal, and this would seem to involve a combination of classical, avoidance, and operant factors—the latter coming into play in relation to the secondary reinforcements the child should receive for not wetting his bed. If these secondary reinforcements are not, at least intermittently, forthcoming, the staying-dry behavior may well undergo extinction so that the innate competing response once again becomes prepotent, thus resulting in a relapse. For this reason it is important to reinforce dry nights either by such social reinforcement as praise or such self-reinforcement as pride of accomplishment. This can be furthered if, as Lovibond (1964) suggests, the child is an active partner in the treatment plan, helping with the essential record keeping and receiving praise for his progress.

Since relapse is not found in all children whose enuresis is treated by conditioning methods, it is possible that those for whom relapse is recorded represent a different population of enuretics. As pointed out in Chapter 8, children who are enuretic can be divided into two groups: one composed of those who had never been dry at night and the other containing those who had once learned to sleep through the night without wetting but regressed to the innate response in later years. In the first group, treatment would consist of teaching a new response not previously available. In the second group, where one is dealing with children for whom an adaptive response had undergone extinction, a previously learned response must be relearned. It would stand to reason that the two groups should differ not only in acquisition rate but also in the resistance to extinction of the response pattern being established in the course of treatment.

Some support for the above speculation comes from a study by Novick (1966) who treated 22 chronic and 23 regressed enuretics by a symptom-focused form of supportive therapy, followed—for those who failed to improve (80 percent)—by a conditioning technique, using a wetting-alarm apparatus. With this combination of treatments, all but 4 of the subjects reached the cure-criterion of 14 consecutive dry nights. Novick reports that the regressed enuretics, that is, those who had acquired enuresis after an initial period of dryness, had reached the cure-criterion sooner and with more rapid decrease in wetting. This would suggest that those who merely had to reestablish a previously learned response learned more quickly than those who had to acquire an entirely new response. On the other hand, the regressed cases were also more likely than the chronic cases to display relapse or new problems, as revealed by follow-up interviews extending over a period of 1 year. It may well be that the relapsing cases reported in other studies are also primarily those for whom enuresis represents a regression. There may be at least two explanations for this phenomenon. The first is that the regressed children reach an acceptable level of dryness sooner than the chronic, thus receiving fewer reinforced training trials with concomitant instability of the adaptive response. Further—and often quickly successful—courses of treatment would thus increase the number of training trials and more firmly establish the desired response. Indeed, DeLeon and Mandell (1966) reported this to be the case. The second (and related) explanation of the relapse phenomenon would seem to lie in the reinforcement contingencies that operate in the regressed child's environment. These may be such that the response of wetting or other maladaptive behavior is more strongly reinforced than the adaptive responses involved in staying dry. This might explain why these children not only regressed originally but relapsed after apparently successful treatment. Therapists would thus do well to work not only with the child but also with the parents who manage the crucial contingencies.

When a problem, such as enuresis, is resolved by a problem-focused approach, traditional therapists, viewing the problem as a symptom of underlying difficulties, make the prediction that the mere removal of one "symptom" will "predispose the child to future symptom formation" (Kessler, 1966, p. 385). Novick (1966) reported that many of his improved subjects developed new symptoms, but it is difficult to evaluate this finding in the absence of a no-treatment control group. Furthermore, the observation is irrelevant to the question of symptom substitution in *behavior therapy* inasmuch as Novick confounded supportive and conditioning treatments.

A study by Baker (1967) was addressed directly to the question of symptom substitution. He treated 10 enuretic children with a conditioning device and compared treatment outcome with equal numbers of children in a no-treatment, waiting list control and a group that received a control treatment, duplicating the waking up and all other aspects of the conditioning treatment, except the conditioning procedure itself. The conditioning group showed significantly more improvement than either control group, and with most of the children in the wakeup group eventually shifted to conditioning, the overall cure rate was 74 percent, another 15 percent showing very marked improvement. Four of the cured subjects relapsed during a 6-months follow-up, but when 2 of these underwent a second course of treatment, they became dry again. In order to investigate the question of symptom substitution and generalization of improvement, an interviewer who did not know to which group a given child had been assigned obtained measures of the child's adjustment from the parents and teachers of the child and from the child himself. These data revealed no symptom substitution, but the cured children showed improvements in areas such as peer relations, school behavior, and general adjustment even though none of these had been directly treated. There was no instance of a worsening of the child's general adjustment.

The bell-and-pad method, which is derived from the respondent conditioning paradigm, is the most frequently used but not the only form of behavior therapy for enuretic children. Several studies report training methods that are explicitly based on the operant model. Hundziak, Maurer, and Watson (1965) made candy, paired with light and tone stimuli, contingent on elimination in the commode. Eight mentally retarded boys between the ages of seven and fourteen, with IQs ranging from 8 to 33, underwent such training. They showed a significantly greater increase in appropriate toilet use than a comparison group of boys who were trained by conventional techniques. The training had been conducted in a special cottage, but once the appropriate responses had been established they generalized to the boys' original living unit. Similar success was reported by Giles and Wolf (1966) who toilet trained 5 severely retarded males through the application of operant conditioning methods.

The work of Giles and Wolf (1966) serves to underscore the importance of finding and using a suitable reinforcer for each child. What is reinforcing for one child may be aversive for the next, and only a careful assessment can assure reinforcer effectiveness. One boy in the Giles and Wolf group refused candy but accepted baby food; others considered a ride in a wheelchair, taking a shower, or returning to bed worthwhile rewards. These authors also found that training could be improved by combining positive reinforcement of the desired response with the delivery of aversive stimuli following the changeworthy inappropriate behavior. When exhaustive use of positive reinforcement had failed to produce results, they introduced punishment consisting of physical restraint. Since this restraint could be removed when appropriate toilet behavior was emitted, it came to serve as a negative reinforcer in addition to its aversive function at the point of introduction. This combination of operant techniques resulted in all these severely retarded children's consistently using the toilet for elimination.

A combination of positive and negative consequences was also used by Gelber and Meyer (1965) who treated a fourteen-year-old boy with an IQ of 117 whose chronic encopresis and fecal smearing were reported to be his only problem behaviors. After hospitalizing the boy in order to gain contingency control, the therapist made time off the ward the reinforcer for appropriate toilet behavior. By introducing an aversive condition (being confined to a hospital ward) which could be terminated following a desired response, negative reinforcement was possible, while punishment for undesirable responses could be introduced by limiting time off the ward and restricting the privilege of walking around the hospital grounds.

Language Deficiencies

While lack of age-appropriate sphincter control is a social handicap, a deficit more crucial to social adaptation is the absence of or gross deficiency in language, such as is frequently encountered in autistic children. The highly complex behavior we call language can be analyzed in operant terms (Skinner, 1957). Accordingly, a word or words emitted by the child are reinforced by the social environment. This paradigm has served as the basis for therapeutic techniques wherein reinforcements are made contingent on the production of sounds or words, and by this method therapists have succeeded in establishing speech in nonverbal or echolalic children. Because a response must occur before it can be reinforced, the child must actively participate in the treatment. The therapist can do little to elicit a word, and when a child is completely nonverbal, speech must be shaped by using any available vocalization and reinforcing successive approximations of language. In some instances (Risley & Wolf, 1967), the child's echolalic behavior can be used as a starting point, while in others (Hewett, 1965; Schell, Stark, & Giddan, 1967) training in social imitation or the therapist's prompts or both must precede speech training (Lovaas, 1966).

Like many children with as gross a disorder as absence of speech, Peter, the four-and-a-half-year-old boy treated by Hewett (1965), manifested other deviant behaviors that interfered with attempts to develop language. His high distractibility and low attention span made it necessary to train him in a specially constructed booth that not only reduced extraneous stimuli but also permitted the introduction of isolation and darkness contingent upon inappropriate responses. Appropriate responses were reinforced with candy and light, but these artificial reinforcers were soon supplemented by the natural reinforcers dispensed by the social environment when a child engages in acceptable and nonaversive behavior. Peter had acquired a 32-word vocabulary after 6 months of speech training, and after a further 8 months, his speaking vocabulary had grown to 150 words, the beginnings of spoken language. During the latter part of training, generalization to the natural environment was stressed—the boy's parents participating in the program. It is significant that Peter's change in behavior altered the reactions of others toward him. The nursing staff came to seek him out for verbal interaction, giving him cues for imitation and insisting on speech before granting requests. Generalization of appropriate speech from the therapy setting to the child's own environment can be enhanced if the therapist sees to it that speech is reinforced under a variety of conditions. Risley and Wolf (1967) have suggested that the child be trained to respond appropriately to a variety of individuals and in a variety of settings, including his own home or the family car.

Early Infantile Autism

The reinforcement value of such social stimuli as praise and approval represent the learning of a generalized reinforcer. Children with severe psychological disorders have frequently failed to acquire this secondary reinforcer so that therapists wishing to strengthen desirable behaviors must resort to the use of such primary reinforcers as food *in the initial stages of treatment*. This obviously limits the situations in which learning can take place to those where food can be readily dispensed and requires that the child be in a state of relative deprivation so that food will be an effective reinforcer. For these reasons, an early therapeutic task with such severely disturbed children as those classified under early infantile autism is the establishment of generalized social reinforcers which can be delivered at any time and are readily available in the child's environment. Ferster (1967) has pointed to the distinction between arbitrary and natural reinforcers. A natural reinforcer is one that the child's environment delivers in spontaneous reaction to his behavior, and when this behavior is adaptive, these natural reinforcers will maintain the behavior in a variety of situations. Once social reinforcers have acquired effectiveness, they will serve to maintain behavior even after the artificial reinforcers used in the beginning stages of treatment have been withdrawn by gradual fading. Patterson, Jones, Whittier, and Wright (1965) have advanced the hypothesis "that the importance of any change in behavior lies in the effect which it produces upon the reactions of the social culture," and it is this reaction which serves to maintain adaptive behavior.

Lovaas, Freitag, Kinder et al. (1966) focused on the establishment of social reinforcers in their work with 2 four-year-old identical twins, who were described as showing "marked autistic features." Following the classical conditioning paradigm, they paired the delivery of food with the social stimulus "good," but despite several hundred trials, this word did not acquire secondary reinforcement properties. When training was shifted to the operant model whereby the presence of the social stimulus came to signal availability of food, these investigators succeeded in establishing the word "good" as a discriminative stimulus. These conditions required that the child attend to the social stimulus, and once this was accomplished, it was possible to use the social stimulus alone as a reinforcer for a simple operant response. As long as the social stimulus continued to be discriminative for food on an intermittent schedule, it retained its acquired reinforcement property over an extended period of time.

This significant study highlights the fact that an event in a child's environment is not a stimulus unless the child attends to the event. It may be that autistic children have difficulty attending to more than one aspect of a stimulus complex at a time, as was suggested in the study by Lovaas, Schreibman, Koegel, and Rehm (1971) which we discussed in Chapter 4. If this were the case, the success of the operant approach, where the respondent approach had failed, might be due to the fact that in the respondent situation, unconditioned and conditioned stimuli occur almost simultaneously and may thus be a stimulus complex, as far as the child is concerned. In the operant situation, on the other hand, discriminative and reinforcing stimuli are temporally separated by the emission of the response, conceivably making it easier for the autistic child to learn under these conditions. In treating autistic children it is important to take their difficulty in attending into consideration. In fact, attention itself might be viewed as a response that can be established through training based on an operant approach (Marr, Miller, & Straub, 1966).

Some behavior will disrupt the acquisition of new and adaptive responses because it is incompatible with learning or with the response that is to be acquired. A child who attends to stimuli other than those presented by the therapist (distractibility) or who makes repetitive and excess responses (hyperactivity) engages in behavior that must be brought under control before treatment can progress. Risley and Wolf (1967) were able to eliminate disruptive behavior by using *time-out from positive reinforcement* (TO). Working on the development of speech in echolalic children, these experimenters found distractibility and hyperactivity to interfere with the training process. They brought mildly disruptive behavior under control by simply looking away until the child once again sat quietly in his chair. More severe forms of disruptive behavior were dealt with by having the therapist leave the room for a set period. The therapist, reentered the room only when the child had not engaged in the disruptive behavior for a short length of time. The therapist's coming back into the room thus served as a negative reinforcer for desired behavior since being alone was an aversive condition for the child, a condition that was being terminated contingent on the behavior to be reinforced.

Operant techniques appear well suited for establishing rather complex behavior repertoires, as has been demonstrated in a number of successful attempts to treat autistic children (Davison, 1964, 1965; Wetzel, Baker, Roney, & Martin, 1966; Lovaas, Schaeffer, Benson, & Simmons, 1965; Wolf, Risley, & Mees, 1964; Wolf, Risley, Johnston, Harris, & Allen, 1967; Brown, Pace, & Becker, 1969).

Deficient Academic and Social Skills

School-age children who are nonreaders manifest a behavioral deficit that calls for the establishment of missing responses. Operant techniques have been applied in a number of studies dealing with such cases. To consider learning to read as operant discrimination learning it is necessary to view the learning task as one in which the child emits the correct verbal response while looking at the written stimulus—the response being followed by some form of reinforcement which, for the accomplished reader, is the information one receives by reading. It is not necessary to make assumptions about the nature of covert cognitive processes in order to plan a training program along these lines. Thus, Staats and Butterfield (1965) applied operant principles to the treatment of a fourteen-year-old boy with a long history of school failures and delinquencies. He was reading at second-grade level when treatment began. Following 40 hours of training, he not only read at the 4.3 grade level but also passed all of his courses for the first time, and his misbehavior in school had completely dropped out. This case not only demonstrated once again that improvement generalizes to areas not specifically designated as treatment targets but it also illustrates how artificial, extrinsic reinforcers (in this case money) can be gradually withdrawn as reading itself becomes reinforcing and other sources of reinforcement come into play to maintain the newly established behavior.

When reading is defined as making the correct verbal response to a particular written stimulus, it can be readily monitored. This, however, is not the case in silent reading where only subsequent changes in performance permit one to infer that reading has taken place. The boy in the Staats and Butterfield (1965) study had been reinforced for silent reading, and, as these authors point out, there is the danger of reinforcing the behavior of just looking at a printed page when no actual reading is going on. A double contingency was introduced in an attempt to guard against this possibility. Several levels of reinforcers (tokens representing different amounts of money) were used so that for looking at a page, a low-value token was presented, while higher-value reinforcers were made contingent on correctly answering questions about the content of the reading material. Unfortunately, the design used here still does not permit an unequivocal answer to the question whether the boy was attending to the printed words instead of merely staring at them because the questions he had to answer were based on the story used for silent reading which had previously been the material for oral reading. This makes it barely conceivable that he had learned the answers to the questions during the readily monitored oral phase after which he did no more than sit and look at the story when he presumably engaged in silent reading.

A flexible use of reinforcement schedules in the course of training is also illustrated in a study by Hewett, Mayhew, and Rabb (1967), who taught basic reading skills to mentally retarded, neurologically impaired, emotionally disturbed, and autistic children. During the first three lessons, reinforcement was on a continuous basis, with one unit of reinforcement for each correct response. After this, each child had to make 5 correct responses before receiving one unit of reinforcement (a 1 to 5 fixed ratio schedule). Reinforcements were such tangibles as candy or money at this point, but in addition, the experimenters began to phase in a token reward in the form of marks on a card, given on a 1 to 1 ratio schedule. The tangible reinforcers were later placed on a 1 to 10 schedule, and ultimately, 200 check marks were needed before they could be exchanged for 1 tangible reinforcer; a 1 to 200 schedule with a delay until the end of the session was thus in operation.

Deficient social skills and complex social behaviors have also been treated by the application of operant principles. Thus, Lovaas, Freitas, Nelson, and Whalen (1967) and Metz (1965) established imitative behavior in schizophrenic children for whom the ability to imitate an adult was a necessary first step toward later acquisition of such socially adaptive behavior as playing games, taking care of personal hygiene, and engaging in appropriate sex-role behavior. Metz (1965) found that imitation generalized to tasks for which specific imitation training had not been given, lending support to the formulation advanced by Gewirtz and Stingle (1968) according to which imitation is a response class that can be learned like other responses.

The deficiency in social skills which is frequently a characteristic of the juvenile delinquent can be dealt with through the application of operant principles as was demonstrated by the work of Schwitzgebel (1964, 1967), who recruited 48 male adolescent delinquents from city streets and provided differential reinforcement for positive statements and constructive behavior, such as prompt arrival at work, that would make the youths more employable. Reinforcements took the form of verbal praise and small gifts which were delivered on a variable ratio schedule, while the subject talked into a tape recorder. This procedure resulted in a significant increase in the number of positive statements, and an improvement in punctuality of arrival for those subjects who had been specifically reinforced for these behaviors. A series of interviews within an operant conditioning framework thus led to dependable and prompt attendance and similar prosocial behaviors in a group that has been notoriously unresponsive to nearly all other forms of treatment.

Other applications of operant principles to work with delinquents are reported by Fineman (1968), Bednar, Zelhart, Greathouse, and Weinberg (1970), and Brown and Tyler (1968). One of the demonstrations of operant technology that is most significant because of its focus on early intervention in delinquency was reported by Phillips, Phillips, Fixsen, and Wolf (1971). Working in a community-based, family-style behavior modification center called Achievement Place, these investigators modified the behavior of six "pre-delinquent" boys, building such social skills as promptness, self-care, saving money, and interest in current events through the use of a token reinforcement procedure in which a child earns points that he can use to obtain privileges or other desirable back-up reinforcers.

Many of the investigators mentioned above use people with relatively little or no professional training as therapeutic agents. In a field where trained professional therapists are in critically short supply, the possibility of using nonprofessional helpers to carry out the treatment program offers exciting potential. We shall return to this issue in the next chapter after we have discussed treatment approaches in cases of excess behavior.

14

TREATMENT APPROACHES – II

When a given behavior occurs with excessive frequency, intensity, or magnitude or where a response is emitted under conditions a child's environment considers inappropriate, the therapeutic task is to bring the behavior within the range of acceptability. Unlike the child with a behavior deficit, who has to learn a response that is not in his repertoire, the child with excess behavior has to learn to modify existing responses. To facilitate this, the therapist has a choice among a variety of techniques which he can use singly or in combination.

PROBLEMS OF EXCESS BEHAVIOR

When treating a child whose problem revolves around excess behavior, the therapist can strengthen responses that are incompatible with the maladaptive response (counterconditioning), withdraw reinforcement (extinction), introduce aversive consequences (punishment), modify setting events preceding the response in question (stimulus deprivation or satiation), or have the child observe appropriate behavior emitted by another (modeling). The choice of therapeutic approach will depend not only on the nature of the target behavior to be modified and the stimuli which maintain it but also on the circumstances under which the child manifests the problem behavior and the aspects of the environment which are subject to the therapist's influences.

Excess Avoidance Responses

Avoidance responses maintained by fear reduction may take a great many forms, but among children one of the most maladaptive is the refusal to attend school, usually called *school phobia*. This may entail either fear of school or fear of leaving home, and only the former is, strictly speaking, a school phobia. Behavior as complex as refusal to attend school has components of both respondent and operant nature, for while the avoidance may have served fear-reducing functions at one time, it is likely that it is later maintained and complicated by the reinforcements available in the home for a child who is not going to school. Many cases of school phobia thus become difficult to treat once the behavior has a long reinforcement history. This consideration led Kennedy (1965) to develop a rapid treatment procedure for children with sudden school phobia of recent onset (Type I, see Chapter 10).

Kennedy's (1965) procedure has six essential components:

1. Good communication with referral sources so that children can be referred on the second or third day after onset of school refusal

2. A deemphasis of somatic complaints with

3. Decisive insistence on school attendance, including the use of force, where necessary

4. A structured, success-focused interview with the parents, stressing the need for a matter-of-fact approach to the problem and the importance of complimenting the child for his going to school and staying there, no matter how brief or stormy that attendance

5. A brief interview with the child, held after school hours in which the importance of going on in the face of fear and the transitory nature of a phobia are stressed

6. An informal telephone follow-up

Using this approach over a period of 8 years, Kennedy treated a total of fifty carefully selected cases, all of whom responded with complete remission. Follow-up failed to reveal evidence for the emergence of other problems, and the children continued to attend school.

The decisive insistence on school attendance emphasized in Kennedy's approach seeks to reduce the possibility of confounding and complicating the school refusal by such factors as the reinforcement involved in staying home, the added source of school avoidance stemming from the missed lessons, which might introduce fear of potential failure upon return to school, and the impossibility of having the fear undergo extinction when the usual condition for extinction—unreinforced exposure to the conditioned stimulus—cannot occur. This last point bears on the self-perpetuating aspects of avoidance responses which are maintained by fear reduction.

Theoretically, a fear response is acquired when a previously neutral stimulus, such as the school building, acquires fear-arousing properties through pairing with a stimulus that, innately or through prior conditioning, has the capacity to elicit fear. This respondent conditioning paradigm—the pairing of an unconditioned stimulus with a conditioned stimulus resulting in a conditioned response—would predict that without further pairing the conditioned response will undergo extinction. Contrary to this prediction, the fear continues and the avoidance response is maintained. What maintains it, as Baum (1966) and Solomon and Brush (1956) have pointed out, is the reinforcing effect of fear reduction contingent on the avoidance response. This protects the child from exposure to the conditioned stimulus, unpaired with the unconditioned stimulus, so that the fear does not undergo extinction. To bring about extinction of a fear response thus maintained, one has to prevent the avoidance response and thereby assure that the child is exposed to the conditioned stimulus but not to the unconditioned stimulus. Such prevention of the avoidance response leads to rapid extinction (Baum, 1966), and Kennedy's (1965) approach to school phobia may well entail aspects of this procedure.

The principles of forced exposure to fear-arousing conditioned stimuli have been incorporated in "implosive therapy" (Stampfl & Levis, 1967) which Smith and Sharpe (1970) used in the treatment of a school-phobic thirteen-year-old boy who had been absent from school for 7 weeks. In implosive therapy, the client is instructed to visualize a highly anxiety-arousing scene involving his phobia: a step intended to expose him in imagery to the conditioned stimulus, unpaired with the unconditioned stimulus. With this procedure Smith and Sharpe were able to have the boy return to his most anxiety-arousing class after one treatment session and to have him in full school attendance after four sessions. They report that the boy continued to attend school thereafter and that his grades and peer relations improved.

Implosive therapy can only be used if a child is highly motivated for help since his cooperation in visualizing fear-arousing situations is absolutely essential. The more frequently used conditioning method for treating fears—counterconditioning as it is involved in systematic desensitization—is less stressful and thus probably more suitable and preferable in work with children.

Garvey and Hegrenes (1966) report the treatment of a school-phobic child by a modified form of desensitization. The therapist and the child approached the school together in a series of steps graded from the least anxiety-evoking situation (sitting in a car in front of the school) to the most anxiety-evoking condition (being in the classroom with the teacher and other students). The authors view this approach as similar to that used by Wolpe (1958) and formulate it in terms of the respondent conditioning paradigm. This, as Lazarus, Davison, and Polefka (1965) have pointed out, overlooks the fact that both respondent and operant factors are at work. Clearly, the therapist's implicit and explicit approval of approach responses reinforces and strengthens such behavior and thus contributes to the treatment.

Conditioning methods have been used in the treatment of

children's fears from the days Mary Cover Jones (1924a) reported her pioneering study with Peter. She reduced this child's fear of furry objects by gradually strengthening fear-incompatible responses, a method that has since come to be known as counterconditioning, systematic desensitization, or therapy by reciprocal inhibition. Relaxation is the fear-incompatible response most frequently used in work with adolescents (Hallsten, 1965) and adults (Wolpe, 1969), but this is only rarely applied in work with children (Tasto, 1969), possibly because training in deep muscle relaxation is difficult with young subjects. For this reason, Lazarus and Abramovitz (1965) explored the use of "emotive imagery," an approach that is based on the assumption that it is possible to inhibit anxiety by the induction of child-appropriate imagery with positive emotional content. Images that presumably serve an anxiety-inhibiting function are those that arouse such feelings as self-assertion, pride, affection, mirth, or fearlessness. The child is instructed to imagine a situation associated with such a feeling, and once such imagery is induced, the therapist presents anxiety-eliciting images, carefully graded from mildly to highly anxiety arousing. On each step on this previously established anxiety hierarchy, the pleasant imagery is paired with anxiety-arousing stimuli, and when treatment is successful, the child should be able to make his fear-incompatible emotional response when the previously anxiety-arousing situation is presented in imagery and, presumably, in real life.

Lazarus and Abramovitz (1965) report success with the method of emotive imagery, but since no systematic research on this approach has been published, there remain many untested assumptions. It is, for example, unknown whether the positive imagery is accompanied by a physiological state that is incompatible with fear, as the notion of reciprocal inhibition would suggest, nor is it known whether verbally presented imagery stimuli do indeed result in a CS pairing, as would be demanded by the respondent conditioning model that is supposed to underly this approach. "Emotive imagery" has interesting implications, but its assumptions remain untested and its claim to efficacy is based on a few clinical reports which lack even rudimentary controls.

A variation of desensitization therapy was used in a case

reported by Straughan (1964). An eight-year-old girl was referred by her mother because the child "was not as happy as she should be." Vaguely worded, general complaints of this nature can usually be broken down into more discrete maladaptive response classes by asking such questions as "What does she *do* that makes you say that she is not happy?" This case was no exception. Further investigation revealed that the child was inhibiting much age-appropriate spontaneous emotional expression in the presence of the mother. Treatment was therefore directed at desensitizing the child to her mother, who had come to be an anxiety-eliciting stimulus. The method used was to have the child in the playroom and to introduce the mother into the girl's presence when she was happily and enthusiastically engaged in play. After five play sessions, the child had indeed learned to be relaxed in the mother's presence and the mother, in turn, was able to learn to interact with the child in a natural and spontaneous manner.

In both implosive and desensitization therapy, the child himself is exposed to the feared stimulus, either in imagery or in real life. When modeling is the treatment of choice, exposure to the feared object is vicarious in that the child merely observes someone else who is making approach responses. A report by Bandura, Grusec, and Menlove (1967) showed that, after having observed a peer model fearlessly make progressively stronger approach responses toward a dog, children who had displayed fearful avoidance behavior toward dogs showed stable and generalized reduction in such behavior. It is possible to present fearless models by means of motion pictures, and the effect on the observer is enhanced if several models display the fearless behavior (Bandura & Menlove, 1968). Ritter (1968) has shown that it is possible to use modeling procedures with groups of children whose snake phobias were treated in this manner.

Since fearful children are constantly exposed to fearless peer models, one might expect that their fears should be reduced in the course of everyday life. While this may well happen with some children, research on modeling suggests why this is not the case in every instance. Observational learning is enhanced when the model resembles the observer. A fearless peer differs from a fearful observer along the dimension of fear. This lack of similarity between model and observer may well attenuate the effectiveness of the observation.

Hill, Liebert, and Mott (1968) report that fear reduction through modeling is made more likely if the model is shown as initially fearful, only gradually emitting fearless approach responses. These investigators produced a film showing an elementary school boy who fearlessly interacted with a dog during the opening scenes and an initially fearful boy of nursery school age who gradually learned to emulate the model's behavior. The sequence thus not only portrayed two models but it also modeled the act of imitation itself. The film was shown once to a group of nine nursery school boys who would not fully approach a harmless caged dog during a pretest. After this single exposure to the film, eight of the children were willing to approach, feed, and pet the large dog, whereas only three of the nine boys in a matched control group were able to do so.

Avoidance responses maintained by fear reduction will often reduce a child's interaction with his social environment, making him appear withdrawn. Withdrawal, however, may also be maintained by its social consequences, in which case removing or changing these consequences should lead to a change in the withdrawn behavior. In many instances, the reinforcing consequence of excessive withdrawal is the attention such behavior calls to itself. It has been repeatedly demonstrated that the selective use of adults' attention can be used to modify problem behaviors of nursery school children, including regressed crawling (Harris et al., 1965), isolate behavior (Allen et al., 1965), and excessive crying and whining (Hart et al., 1965). In each of these studies, adult attention was withheld from the target behavior and made contingent on behavior that was incompatible with it. To test the efficacy of this manipulation, the contingencies were experimentally reversed with a resulting recurrence of the maladaptive behavior, demonstrating that adult attention was indeed the independent variable responsible for the behavior modification. Following this experimental reversal, the therapeutic contingencies are obviously reinstated so that the end result of the intervention is adaptive behavior on the part of the child.

Excess Approach Behavior

The principles of reinforcement which have been successfully applied in the modification of relatively simple cases of avoidance behavior of nursery school children have also been used to good effect in cases of complex, multiple problems involving temper tantrums, difficult peer relations, and negativism (Patterson & Brodsky, 1966); stuttering (Browning, 1967; Rickard & Mundy, 1965); excessive scratching (Allen & Harris, 1966); and high-frequency self-stimulatory behavior (Koegel & Covert, 1972). Disruptive classroom behavior has been reduced by instructing teachers to shift their reinforcing attention to desirable alternative behaviors (Thomas, Becker, & Armstrong, 1968) and by introducing a token reinforcement program (O'Leary & Becker, 1967; O'Leary, Becker, Evans, & Saudargas, 1969).

Patterson (1965) and Patterson, Jones, Whittier, and Wright (1965) reduced hyperactivity in school children by selectively reinforcing periods during which such nonattending behaviors as arm and leg movements, shuffling of chair, looking out of window, fiddling, talking to self, and wiggling of feet did not occur. The treatment made reinforcement contingent on the "non-occurrence of non-attending behavior," a method known as differential reinforcement of other behavior (DRO). The formulation involving the double negative is dictated by the need to focus on observable behavior. It is possible to keep an objective, reliable record of such behaviors as fingering a box of crayons, while it is not possible to observe "paying attention" in any direct manner. In work of this nature, it is customary and desirable to announce the reinforcement contingencies to the child, and in Patterson's studies, not only the hyperactive child but also the entire class was told that the aim of the procedure was to help him sit still so that he could study better. The class was told that when the boy sat still, he would earn candy for himself and the rest of the children in the room. This reduced the amount of distraction offered by the classmates and, in one case (Patterson, 1965), led to clapping and cheering at the end of a trial—social reinforcement delivered by the peer group.

Spelling out contingencies would seem to be an obvious procedure when working with a child in therapy. But to the psychologist with a background in laboratory conditioning studies, it represents an unusual procedure, since in laboratory work with humans, instructions of this kind would confound the experiment, making it impossible to ascertain whether a newly established response is a function of the independent variable under investigation or the result of the subject's compliance with the experimenter's stated intentions. As long as it is necessary to test the effectiveness of a specific therapeutic procedure, a verbal statement of the contingencies announced to the client would indeed confound the experiment, but where a therapeutic program has advanced beyond the experimental stage, anything that enhances the treatment process—be that a placebo effect or verbal instructions—ought to be brought to bear in helping the client.

It was around this point that Doubros and Daniels (1966) took issue with Patterson's approach of announcing the contingencies to the child and his classmates. They felt that this introduces uncontrolled social reinforcement and awareness, factors they attempted to control in their own work on the reduction of hyperactivity in six mentally retarded boys. As a result of their controlled experiment, it is now possible to state that differential reinforcement of other behavior (DRO) can be an effective method for reducing hyperactivity and increasing constructive play. On the other hand, Doubros and Daniels carried out their work in a playroom where each child was treated by himself so that it is not known whether the responses they learned there generalized to other settings.

Where complex behavior or behavior patterns must be modified, a combination of treatment methods may be required, and the manipulation of only one reinforcement contingency may not be sufficient to bring about the desired changes. The case of Dicky, reported by Wolf, Risley, and Mees (1964) and Wolf et al. (1967) serves to illustrate the use of a combination of techniques, including the manipulation of a variety of contingencies in conditioning and extinction procedures and the introduction of a form of aversive control in order to reduce the frequency of grossly maladaptive behavior. Dicky was three-and-a-half years old and had been diagnosed as a case of childhood schizophrenia. He engaged in such self-destructive behaviors as head banging, hair pulling, face slapping, and scratching. He lacked adaptive social and verbal repertoires, refused to sleep alone, and did not eat in an age-appropriate fashion. His case became critical because he was in danger of losing his eyesight. Because of cataracts in both eyes, he had to have surgical removal of the lenses, and since he refused to wear glasses and habitually threw them on the floor, permanent retinal damage was very likely.

The therapists first attacked the boy's refusal to wear his eyeglasses because that seemed the most serious, immediate problem. Glasses wearing was gradually established by reinforcing it with food and later on with opportunities to take walks, go on rides, or play. Because the child's glasses-throwing behavior was incompatible with glasses wearing, a mild form of punishment was made contingent on glasses throwing. Following each glasses-throw, Dicky was put in his room for 10 minutes, a form of time-out from positive reinforcement (TO), if one views being in the company of others as a positively reinforcing condition. The same TO method was used to eliminate tantrums, self-slapping, and the pinching of teachers and other children in the nursery school. The effectiveness of this technique was demonstrated by experimental reversal (Wolf, Risley, & Mees, 1964). Glasses-throwing had taken place at the rate of approximately two times per day before treatment was initiated. Within 5 days of instituting the TO procedure, the rate of this behavior had decreased to zero, but when Dicky was no longer put in his room for throwing the glasses, thus reversing the contingencies, the rate of glasses-throwing returned to its original high level after about 3 weeks. When Dicky was once again put in his room whenever this behavior occurred, it quickly decreased in frequency and virtually disappeared within 6 days.

Reversal in applied behavior analysis permits one to evaluate the reliability of a treatment procedure for an individual subject (Baer, Wolf, & Risley, 1968). The first step in this analysis is to record the behavior in question and to examine the record over time until the stability of the measure is established. After a record of the base line is thus obtained, the particular contingency is introduced, and the behavior continues to be measured and recorded in order to ascertain whether the experimental (treatment) variable produces a behavior change. If such a change occurs, the contingency is altered or discontinued, and if the behavioral change does indeed depend on it, this change should be lost or diminished (hence, "reversal"). Following this, the experimental variable is once again applied to see if the behavior change can be reinstated. If it can, the contingency in question continues to be used inasmuch as it has been demonstrated through one or more of such reversal procedures that it is a reliable treatment method. In many instances such a demonstration serves not the esoteric scientific interest of the behavior therapist but is necessary in order to convince a child's parents, teachers, or institutional attendants of the efficacy of the approach inasmuch as their cooperation in contingency management is often an essential aspect of the treatment plan.

Reversal can only be carried out if the target behavior is carefully defined and objectively measured, but the need for such measurement goes beyond the requirements of behavior analysis and education, for without it, treatment becomes unsystematic and outcome impossible to define. This is illustrated in further work with Dicky, as reported by Wolf, Risley, Johnston, Harris, and Allen (1967). After some of his more bizarre behavior had been modified during hospitalization, Dicky was enrolled in a nursery school where he emitted a high rate of pinching teachers and other children. At first, an attempt was made to put this behavior on an extinction schedule by ignoring it, but when this failed to change the pinching rate, Dicky was sent to a specially set aside small room whenever pinching occurred. After the first use of this time-out contingency, the rate of pinching decreased drastically, only 4 more instances of it being recorded over the next 74 class sessions. Prior to the introduction of the TO procedure, a teacher had attempted to modify the pinching by reinforcing patting, which was seen as an incompatible alternate response. Patting behavior stabilized at a moderate rate within a few sessions when Dicky was encouraged and praised for emitting this response. At this point, the teachers reported that they were succeeding in replacing pinching by patting. However, the observer's record on which instances of both patting and pinching had been entered for every 10-second interval clearly showed that contrary to the teachers' impression, the pinching rate had not decreased and that it did not decline until the TO procedure was instituted some 13 sessions later. Without the quantitative observer record, the teachers would have been under the mistaken impression that the development of a substitute response had been responsible for the decrease in the objectionable behavior. Inasmuch as Dicky's parents were to be instructed in the use of behavior modification techniques so that they could supplement the treatment at home, such an erroneous conclusion might have contributed to treatment failure and disappointment. With the variety of approaches used in Dicky's case over a period of 3 years, the boy was eventually able to attend a special education class in public school where he made a good adjustment and learned to read at the primary level.

The Use of Negative Consequences

In the case of Dicky it was possible to eliminate such atavistic behaviors as tantrums and self-slapping by the introduction of a relatively mild negative consequence (Time-Out). This, as we shall see, is usually sufficiently potent to bring such behavior under control, but on occasion, particularly with profoundly disturbed children and where self-injurious behavior represents an immediate danger to the child's life, more drastic negative consequences have to be brought to bear before adaptive behavior can be established. It is in those rare instances that the behavior therapist must resort to aversive conditioning (punishment) if the child is to be helped. The chronic ruminative vomiting of some profoundly retarded children, for example, is an instance where death may be the alternative to the drastic intervention which is represented by the use of response contingent, brief electric shock to the thigh or some other part of the body. This has proved effective where other medical and psychological methods had failed (Lang & Melamed, 1969; Luckey, Watson, & Musick, 1968).

Reinforcement theory holds that responses that are consistently and immediately followed by an aversive stimulus (pain) should become suppressed. The self-injurious behavior of such grossly disordered children as Dicky thus represents an apparent paradox because such responses as self-hitting are maintained despite their negative consequences. Some have assumed that the child has a "need" to hurt himself, that he "enjoys" the self-inflicted punishment. If this explanation were correct, then any treatment that involved the introduction of negative consequences contingent on self-injurious behavior should serve to further strengthen such behavior. Yet reports by Wolf, Risley, and Mees (1964) ; Lovaas et al., (1965) ; and Tate and Baroff (1966) vitiate the "masochism" explanation inasmuch as these investigators were able to reduce the incidence of self-injurious behavior by the introduction of aversive consequences (punishment) to such behavior.

The contingencies surrounding self-injurious behavior were analyzed by Lovaas, Freitag, Gold, and Kassorla (1965), who concluded that such behavior is maintained not by the "pleasure" the child gets out of hurting himself but by the social reinforcement entailed in the attention such behavior almost invariably calls to itself. These investigators showed that self-injurious behavior decreases when it is ignored but increases when it is followed by such solicitous, "interpretive" comments as "I don't think you are bad." While effective, the extinction process entailed in ignoring self-injurious behavior is often too slow, and the risk of permanent physical harm frequently demands that the behavior be modified at a more rapid rate. In addition, behavior tends to increase in frequency, intensity, or duration when an extinction schedule is first introduced and before the rate gradually declines. For these reasons, Risley (1968), Tate and Baroff (1966), and Lovaas and his coworkers (1965) stress the rapid response suppression possible when electric shock is made contingent on self-injurious responses, particularly when this approach is combined with the positive reinforcement of incompatible, adaptive behavior.

Physical punishment should be used only when the behavior in question must be quickly suppressed because delay would endanger the child or make the learning of adaptive responses impossible. In the case reported by Risley (1968), for example, the child engaged in climbing behavior that not only endangered her safety but also thwarted all attempts to teach constructive responses. Before introducing punishment with electric shock, Risley had tried time-out procedures, extinction, and reinforcement of incompatible behaviors without success. When punishment seemed the only means left, careful records were kept to assure that it had no undesirable side effects, such as suppressing other behaviors, and the use of shock was discontinued as soon as the target behavior had been brought under control. For less dangerous atavistic behaviors, such as the child's autistic rocking, less severe forms of negative consequences continued to be the method of choice.

In most cases the negative consequences involved in time out from positive reinforcement, such as social isolation or deprivation of privileges, appear sufficiently potent to weaken undesirable responses. Even such ordinarily intractable behavior as the antisocial acts of institutionalized adolescent delinquents can be modified by the use of a 15-minute period of isolation when it is introduced immediately and consistently as a consequence of every instance of specified unacceptable behaviors (Tyler & Brown, 1967, Burchard & Tyler, 1965). Since stealing carries its own inherent reinforcement, it would seem to be particularly difficult to treat, but Wetzel (1966) succeeded in eliminating the stealing behavior of an institutionalized boy by using a time-out procedure. In order to have something that could be withdrawn contingent on the boy's stealing, it was necessary to create a condition of positive reinforcement, in this case the privilege of visiting the cook of the institution. Once these visits had acquired positive reinforcement value, the loss of this privilege became a potent aversive condition.

There appears to be a paradox in the fact that such relatively mild punishment as having to spend 15 minutes in an empty room can effectively modify behavior of delinquents for whom far more severe punishments have usually been ineffective. Burchard and Tyler (1965), for example, succeeded in reducing the antisocial behavior of a 13-year-old, institutionalized delinquent boy through the use of isolation, combined with positive reinforcement for clearly defined periods that he did not have to spend in isolation. Yet this same boy had spent a total of 200 days in an individual isolation room during the year prior to the onset of the reported study, and during that time his behavior had become increasingly unmanageable. The prime difference between the systematic and the unsystematic use of punishment would seem to explain this apparent paradox. In the systematic application of operant principles, negative consequences to unacceptable behavior are *immediately* and *consistently* introduced whenever unacceptable behavior occurs. When punishment is used unsystematically, unacceptable behavior usually has to reach a given magnitude before the adults in the environment intervene, and even then the punishment is usually introduced as a last resort. A great many interpersonal events take place between the incipient onset of the unacceptable behavior and the eventual introduction of the negative consequences, and these events tend to serve a reinforcing and not a suppressing function.

Burchard and Tyler (1965) describe the temporal sequence of staff behavior to the disruptive behavior of one of the boys as follows: When Donny first begins to "act up," staff members try to ignore this behavior for as long as possible. During this time, peer approval and attention tend to reinforce the behavior. As the behavior continues and increases in magnitude, attendants turn to attempts at supportive persuasion to desist. When this (reinforcement) is unsuccessful, the staff becomes angry and only at that point punishment is finally introduced. But that is not all. Staff members now feel guilty, and this reaction manifests itself in sympathy visits to the child in the isolation room. With the contingencies structured in this fashion, it is not surprising that Donny's unacceptable behavior increased over time for staff and peer attention occurred immediately after the response, while the punishment was delayed and ambivalently administered. The time-out program instituted by Burchard and Tyler, on the other hand, had Donny immediately and perfunctorily placed in his isolation room as soon as he displayed any unacceptable behavior. The staff was instructed to approach this intervention in a matter-of-fact way and at the onset of carefully specified target behavior, that is, before they themselves had become emotionally aroused by the behavior. It was also stressed that isolation had to be on an all-or-none basis and that it should never be used as a threat. It is very likely that the systematic nature of punishment when used in the operant frame of reference is the principal factor in its efficiency. In everyday child rearing, punishment tends to be used in the unsystematic, arbitrary, last-resort fashion described by Burchard and Tyler, and this probably explains why it is rarely an effective technique for the suppression of undesirable behavior.

TREATMENT BY NONPROFESSIONALS

Because the operant techniques can be described in relatively simple terms and their application taught in a short time, treatment using these techniques can be carried out by nonprofessional[1] people, working under the direction of a professional person who has expert knowledge of the theoretical basis and works out the details of the treatment plan. It has thus been possible to involve ward attendants (Gardner 1972; Giles & Wolf, 1966), nursery school teachers (Hart et al., 1965), classroom teachers (O'Leary et al., 1969), and parents (Wahler, 1969) in treatment programs. Hawkins et al., (1966); Jensen and Womack (1967); O'Leary, O'Leary, and Becker (1967); Patterson, Ray, and Shaw (1968); Wahler, Winkel, Peterson, and Morrison (1965); and Zeilberger, Sampen, and Sloane (1968) all report the effective use of mothers as behavior therapists for their own children.

If behavior is to be modified, the modification must take place when and where the behavior manifests itself, that is, where the reinforcing contingencies are most likely to be operating. This is rarely the therapist's consulting room. As a consequence, behavior therapists working with children frequently find themselves operating in the "natural environment" (Tharp & Wetzel, 1969) and through adults who are in a position to be present when the target behavior takes place and who have control over the contingencies of reinforcement (Wahler, 1969). In the case of children in schools or institutions, these adults are teachers, nurses, and attendants (Hall, Cristler, Cranston, & Tucker, 1970; Hall et al., 1971). In the case of children living at home, the parents become the logical contingency managers, hence, therapists (Johnson & Brown, 1969). In order to engage parents as the child's actual therapists, it is necessary to train them in the essential techniques, including the essential objective recording (Hirsch, 1968), and in some instances in the ability to discriminate the incipient stages of the objectionable behavior. This was done by Hawkins et al. (1966) who had a mother treat her four-year-old boy who had been extremely difficult to manage and control. He would kick objects and people, tear at his clothing, hit himself, and generally require almost constant attention. At first the mother found it difficult to recognize the incipient stages of the target behavior and to be consistent in her response to it. She was therefore taught by the professional therapist, who entered the home

[1] The term "nonprofessional" is used to denote those who are not members of the traditional "mental health" professions, though they may be members of their own respected professions.

for this purpose, when to use praise, attention, affectionate physical contact, verbal commands, and isolation. This mother quickly learned both the necessary discrimination and the appropriate reactions, thus being able to carry the treatment to successful conclusion.

In Chapter 2 we cited a projection by Miller, Hampe, Barrett, and Noble (1971) according to which there is 1 professional child therapist for every 8,000 troubled children. It is one of the most exciting prospects of behavior therapy that it permits an increase of therapeutic manpower and—through parent education—a potential decrease in the number of troubled children. On this optimistic note we now turn to an examination of available research on the effectiveness of the behavioral approach to the treatment of psychological disorders.

15

THE EFFECTIVENESS
OF BEHAVIOR
THERAPY FOR CHILDREN

No treatment procedure can be said to have demonstrated its effectiveness until the stability of improvements has been analyzed over time. This calls for systematic follow-up studies, but these are exceedingly rare, not only for behavior therapy but for any kind of psychological treatment of disordered behavior. The few exceptions (Baker, 1969; Kennedy, 1965; Nolan, Mattis & Holliday, 1970) suggest that over such relatively short periods as 12 months, improvements attributed to behavior therapy have been maintained. In fact, as both Baker (1969) and Nolan et al. (1970) report, children thus treated often show improvements in areas that had not been specific targets of the behavior therapy. This may be a reflection of the fact that problem behaviors prevent the child from engaging in behavior that might be a source of positive reinforcement for him, reinforcement which becomes available for building an adaptive repertoire once the problem behavior is removed. It is, of course, not possible to say for how long a treated case should be followed before one can speak with confidence about the stability of improvement. Nor would it necessarily be proof of the ineffectiveness of treatment if a former client developed new problems many years after apparently successful treatment. Therapy is not a form of immunization, and an individual may always encounter circumstances under which maladaptive behavior can once again be acquired.

The reasons for the dearth of well-controlled outcome and follow-up studies are well known. As Bergin (1966) and Paul (1967b) have pointed out, it is difficult to meet the requirements of meaningful outcome research. Relevant control groups are hard to find, therapies and therapists are difficult to equate, a sufficient number of cases with the same problem behavior are rarely available, and tracing terminated clients for careful follow-up assessment is time-consuming and expensive.

A problem that lends itself more readily to experimental study than most psychological disorders is bed-wetting. Enuresis is readily operationalized and objectively measured; it has a high enough frequency in the child population to permit a researcher to gather a reasonably large number of subjects in relatively short time. Withholding treatment from an enuretic child for a period of months in order to have him in a control group does not raise major ethical qualms because his problem does not represent a danger to him or others and is unlikely to worsen without immediate treatment. Lastly, the behavioral treatment of enuresis entails a well-developed conditioning technique that requires minimal activity on the part of the therapist so that he can treat a relatively large number of children during a reasonably limited period of time. For all these reasons, the best outcome research available deals with the conditioning treatment of bed-wetting. Such studies (De Leon & Mandell, 1966; Baker, 1969; Lovibond, 1964) have compared conditioning treatment with other modes of therapy and with no-treatment controls. In all instances, the children treated by the bell-and-buzzer conditioning methods reached cure criterion earlier than those treated by other methods or held in the control group.

The effectiveness of a behaviorally oriented treatment for problems in peer relationship was studied by Clement and Milne (1967) who compared such treatment with a more traditional play-therapy approach and with no adult contact. By requesting all third grade teachers in a school district to refer boys who were socially withdrawn, nonspontaneous, and friendless, Clement and Milne obtained

11 children whom they assigned to one of three conditions : a token group, a therapist group, and a control group. The children in the token group participated in 14 weekly 50-minute group-play sessions during which they received tokens as reinforcement for social approach behavior. The therapist group was given the same treatment but without the use of tangible reinforcers, and the control met in the playroom without a therapist while being observed through a one-way mirror.

The dependent variables were measures of productivity, anxiety, social adjustment, general psychological adjustment, and discrete problem behaviors. Some of these measures were based on observations, others on tests and mothers' reports. The analysis of the results showed the token group to have improved on 4 measures, while the therapist group improved on 2 and got worse on 1. The control group did not show any improvement. The measure on which the therapist group deteriorated while the token group improved was social play—the amount of time the children spent playing with each other. Since this had been one of the specifically reinforced behaviors, the finding strengthens the authors' conclusion that operant reinforcement is effective in treating shy, withdrawn eight-year-old boys in a group situation. At the same time it should be pointed out that this study had several weaknesses of which the authors were well aware. The therapist was the same for both groups, and he knew the hypotheses being tested. Some of the measures had low reliability, and the size of the sample was exceedingly small. For these reasons, the results of this study should be interpreted with considerable circumspection, particularly before one generalizes from it to behavior therapy as conducted with a typical clinic population.

What is probably the most massive study of the effectiveness of behavior therapy with severely disturbed children was reported by Lovaas, Koegel, Simmons, and Stevens (1973) who treated 20 autistic children and took careful, reliable, quantitative measures of behavior. These measures reflected self-stimulation, echolalic speech, appropriate speech, social nonverbal behavior, and appropriate play. In addition, data on intelligence test scores and the results from the Vineland Social Maturity Scale were assessed. The authors report that during treatment disordered behavior decreased, while prosocial behavior increased for all 20 children, although the changes were not equally great for all. Some of the children developed spontaneous social interaction and the spontaneous use of language. Intelligence and social quotients showed large gains during treatment. When the same measures were used in a follow-up 2 years after treatment, large differences emerged depending on whether or not the children had been institutionalized at the conclusion of their exposure to behavior therapy. Those children whose parents had been taught to use contingency management in the home continued to improve, while those whose parents had not learned to be their child's behavior therapist but who had been sent to institutions where the contingencies were totally different from those under which the constructive behavior had been learned, regressed and deteriorated.

This report by Lovaas et al. (1973) also mentions the generalization of improvement to areas that had not been specific treatment targets. Thus, children who had been chronic toe-walkers began to walk normally after 4 to 5 months of treatment; those who had never slept through the night began to put in 10 hours of uninterrupted sleep, etc. At the same time, the authors clearly state that their treatment was not a "cure for autism." They made remarkable progress with children for whom other forms of treatment had been ineffective, and they were able to demonstrate that for children whose home environment can take over the treatment program by applying systematic contingency management, dramatic improvement can be recorded.

A comprehensive review of the literature pertaining to the use of behavior therapy with psychotic children was prepared by Leff (1968) who concluded that "behavior-modification techniques may be extremely useful tools in the education and rehabilitation of psychotic children" (p. 406). He points out that none of the investigators whose work he reviewed would claim that they have cured their subjects, but he adds that many could justifiably state that "they have equipped their subjects with several of the basic skills and habits necessary for the most rudimentary of adjustments to their social environment" (ibid.).

While several well-controlled studies (Lang, Lazovik, & Reynolds, 1965; Paul, 1966, 1967a; Paul & Shannon, 1966) have demonstrated the effectiveness of behavior therapy with adults, a great deal of the experimental support for behavior therapy with children comes from studies using the "reversal" design where each subject serves as his own control (e.g., Browning & Stover, 1971; Hart et al., 1965; Hawkins et al., 1966; Wolf & Risley, 1967). This design permits one to demonstrate that the target behavior did not change before the particular intervention was introduced and that changes were correlated with the experimental manipulation of the intervention. The reliable effect of the intervention can thus be shown rather convincingly, but since there is no untreated control group, the question whether the problem would have undergone remission without treatment cannot be addressed. Some reports, such as that published by Burchard and Tyler (1965), show that a given child's behavior did not improve or, in fact, deteriorated under different forms of treatment and that positive changes occurred when a behavioral approach was instituted. Yet even here, it is not clear whether the improvement was a function of the manipulation the investigators introduced, which aspect of the manipulation was the effective component, and whether the change was due to a placebo or "Hawthorne" effect. Other reports, such as that by Patterson, Jones, Whittier, and Wright (1965), compare one experimental child with one control child, thus illustrating the effectiveness of an intervention. But case studies of this nature, though often dramatic, may well represent a selected and biased sample from the total population of treated cases so that they cannot be adduced as evidence for the effectiveness of behavior therapy, let alone for its superiority over other methods.

There exists one unpublished study that is reported to have systematically compared behavior therapy, traditional psychotherapy, and a no-treatment condition using a typical clinic population. It was conducted by James Humphery and is cited by Eysenck (1967). Humphery studied 71 children who had been referred to child guidance clinics for a variety of disorders, excluding those with brain damage and psychosis. These children were divided into 3 groups: A control group of 34 children was evaluated at the beginning and again at the conclusion of the study, receiving no treatment of any kind during that period. Of the remaining children, one group received behavior therapy (desensitization), while the other was given traditional psychotherapy. Evaluation of all children was on a 5-point scale of severity of disorder, "cure" being defined as a rise of 2 or more points on this instrument. Clinicians who did not know to which group a given child had been assigned conducted the evaluations.

Treatment for each case was terminated when the therapist and a consulting psychiatrist decided that maximum benefit had been obtained. By this criterion of termination, the children who had been in psychotherapy received 21 sessions, spread over 31 weeks, while those in behavior therapy received 9 sessions, spread over 18 weeks. On the basis of the criterion measure, 75 percent of the children in behavior therapy were rated as cured at the termination of treatment, compared to 35 percent of those who had been in psychotherapy. Follow-up 10 months later revealed that 85 percent of those who had received behavior therapy were now rated as cured, while only 29 percent of those who had received psychotherapy were still considered to be in that category. Of the no-treatment control group, 18 percent were found to be cured when they were re-evaluated at follow-up.

Several flaws detract from the validity of the conclusions of this study. A 5-point rating scale of severity of difficulty would seem a relatively insensitive instrument with which to detect changes in a child's behavior, and the unusually brief time devoted to psychotherapy raises the question whether that treatment was represented in its most typical form. Furthermore, a bias in sampling had resulted in the assignment of more seriously disturbed children to the behavior therapy group than to the psychotherapy group. The psychotherapy group thus had more favorable ratings at the beginning of treatment, so that a ceiling effect made it less likely for them to achieve the 2-point rise that defined cure. All told, a definitive experimental comparison of behavior therapy and psychotherapy with children, using a typical child guidance population with heterogeneous problems, remains to be carried out.

One might, of course, question the necessity of proving the superiority of one form of treatment over another. There are now many studies which attest to the effectiveness of behavior therapy with the wide variety of problems where it has been applied. There is also no question that behavior therapists reach their defined treatment goal more quickly than psychotherapists reach their criterion for terminating a case. Even if behavior therapy were ultimately to prove to be no more effective than psychotherapy, it is certainly more efficient, in terms of both time and professional effort. Rather than studying the question whether one form of treatment is superior to another, it would seem wiser to investigate what, if anything, are the effective ingredients in various forms of treatment and what kinds of problems are best treated by which method. It is unlikely that behavior therapy as it is practiced today is the panacea for every conceivable psychological disorder. So far, only the conditioning and modeling paradigms have been applied to clinical problems in any systematic fashion. In all probability, other knowledge from the behavioral sciences has relevance to the treatment of psychological disorders, and it is to the gathering and application of such knowledge that future efforts should be directed.

REFERENCES

Achenbach, T. M.
The classification of children's psychiatric symptoms: A factor-analytic study. *Psychological Monographs,* 1966, **80**, 6.

Achenbach, T., & Zigler, E.
Cue-learning and problem-learning strategies in normal and retarded children. *Child Development,* 1968, **39**, 827–848.

Ackerson, L.
Children's behavior problems. Chicago: University of Chicago Press, 1931.

Ackerson, L.
Children's behavior problems: II. Relative importance and interrelations among traits. *Behavior research fund monograph.* Chicago: University of Chicago Press, 1942.

Allen, K. E., & Harris, F. R.
Elimination of a child's excessive scratching by training the mother in reinforcement procedures. *Behaviour Research and Therapy,* 1966, **4**, 79–84.

Allen, K. E., Hart, B. M., Buell, J. S., Harris, F. R., & Wolf, M. M.
Effects of social reinforcement on isolate behavior of a nursery
school child. In L. P. Ullmann & L. Krasner (Eds.), *Case studies in
behavior modification.* New York: Holt, 1965. Pp. 307–312.

Allen, M. K., & Liebert, R. M.
Children's adoption of self-reward patterns: Model's prior experience
and incentive for non-imitation. *Child Development,* 1969, **40,**
921–926. (a)

Allen, M. K., & Liebert, R. M.
Effects of live and symbolic deviant-modeling cues on adoption of a
previously learned standard. *Journal of Personality and Social
Psychology,* 1969, **11,** 253–260. (b)

Anand, B. K.
Nervous regulation of food intake. *Physiological Review,* 1961, **41,**
677–708.

Aronfreed, J., & Reber, A.
Internalized behavioral suppression and the timing of social
punishment. *Journal of Personality and Social Psychology,* 1965, **1,**
3–16.

Ax, A. F.
The physiological differentiation between fear and anger in humans.
Psychosomatic Medicine, 1953, **15,** 433–442.

Baer, D. M., Wolf, M. M., & Risley, T. R.
Some current dimensions of applied behavior analysis. *Journal of
Applied Behavior Analysis,* 1968, **1,** 91–97.

Bailey, J., & Meyerson, L.
Vibration as a reinforcer with a profoundly retarded child. *Journal of
Applied Behavior Analysis,* 1969, **2,** 135–137.

Baker, B. L.
Symptom treatment and symptom substitution in enuresis. *Journal of
Abnormal Psychology,* 1969, **74,** 42–49.

Baldwin, V. L.
Development of social skills in retardates as a function of three types

of reinforcement programs. *Dissertation Abstracts,* 1967, **27**, (9-A), 2865.

Bandura, A.
Psychotherapy as a learning process. *Psychological Bulletin,* 1961, **58**, 143–159.

Bandura, A.
Principles of behavior modification. New York: Holt, 1969.

Bandura, A., Grusec, J. E., & Menlove, F. L.
Vicarious extinction of avoidance behavior. *Journal of Personality and Social Psychology,* 1967, **5**, 16–23.

Bandura, A., & Menlove, F. L.
Factors determining vicarious extinction of avoidance behavior through symbolic modeling. *Journal of Personality and Social Psychology,* 1968, **8**, 99–108.

Bandura, A., & Mischel, W.
Modification and self-imposed delay of reward through exposure to live and symbolic models. *Journal of Personality and Social Psychology,* 1965, **2**, 698–705.

Bandura, A., & Rosenthal, T. L.
Vicarious classical conditioning as a function of arousal level. *Journal of Personality and Social Psychology,* 1966, **3**, 54–62.

Bandura, A., & Walters, R. H.
Adolescent aggression. New York: Ronald, 1959.

Bandura, A., & Walters, R. H.
Aggression. In H. W. Stevenson, J. Kagan, & C. Spiker (Eds.), *Child Psychology, The 62nd Yearbook of the National Society for the Study of Education.* Chicago: National Society for the Study of Education, 1963. Pp. 364–415.

Bateman, B. D. & Schiefelbusch, R. L.
Educational identification, assessment, and evaluation procedures. In *Minimal Brain Dysfunctions in Children,* U. S. Public Health Service Publication No. 2015. Washington, D. C.: U. S. Department of Health, Education and Welfare, 1969. Pp. 5–20.

Baum, M.
Rapid extinction of an avoidance response following a period of response prevention in the avoidance apparatus. *Psychological Reports,* 1966, **18**, 59–64.

Becker, W. C., & Krug, R. S.
A circumplex model for social behavior of children. *Child Development,* 1964, **35**, 371–396.

Becker, W. C., Peterson, D. R., Luria, Z., Shoemaker, D. J., & Hellmer, L. A.
Relations of factors derived from parent-interview ratings to behavior problems in five-year-olds. *Child Development,* 1962, **33**, 509–535.

Bednar, R. L., Zelhart, P. F., Greathouse, L., & Weinberg, S.
Operant conditioning principles in the treatment of learning and behavior problems with delinquent boys. *Journal of Counseling Psychology,* 1970, **17**, 492–497.

Beery, J. W.
Matching of auditory and visual stimuli by average and retarded readers. *Child Development,* 1967, **38**, 827–833.

Bender, L.
Childhood schizophrenia. *American Journal of Orthopsychiatry,* 1947, **17**, 40–56.

Bergin, A. E.
Some implications of psychotherapy research for therapeutic practice. *Journal of Abnormal Psychology,* 1966, **71**, 235–246.

Berkowitz, P. H.
Some psychological aspects of mental illness in children. *Genetic Psychology Monographs,* 1961, **63**, 103–148.

Berlyne, D. E.
Conflict, arousal, and curiosity. New York: McGraw-Hill, 1960.

Bettelheim, B.
The empty fortress. New York: Free Press, 1967.

Bijou, S. W.
A functional analysis of retarded behavior. In N. R. Ellis (Ed.), *International review of research in mental retardation.* Vol. 1. New York: Academic, 1966. Pp. 1–19.

Bindman, S. S.
Personality characteristics of the parents of children diagnosed as schizophrenic. *Dissertation Abstracts,* 1966, **27**, 298–299.

Birch, H. G., & Belmont, L.
Auditory-visual integration in normal and retarded readers. *American Journal of Orthopsychiatry,* 1964, **34**, 852–861.

Birch, H. G., Belmont, L., Belmont, I., & Taft, L. T.
Brain damage and intelligence in educable mentally subnormal children. *Journal of Nervous and Mental Disease,* 1967, **144**, 247–257.

Birnbrauer, J. S.
Preparing "uncontrollable" retarded children for group instruction. Paper presented at the meeting of the American Educational Research Association, 1967.

Birnbrauer, J. S., Bijou, S. W., Wolf, M. M., & Kidder, J. D.
Programed instruction in the classroom. In L. P. Ullmann & L. Krasner (Eds.), *Case studies in behavior modification.* New York: Holt, 1965. Pp. 358–363.

Birnbrauer, J. S., Wolf, M. M., Kidder, J. D., & Tague, C. E.
Classroom behavior of retarded pupils with token reinforcement. *Journal of Experimental Child Psychology,* 1965, **2**, 219–235.

Bliss, E. L., & Branch, C. H. H.
Anorexia nervosa: its history, psychology, and biology. New York: Hoeber-Harper, 1960.

Blitzer, J. R., Rollins, N., & Blackwell, A.
Children who starve themselves: Anorexia nervosa. *Psychosomatic Medicine,* 1961, **23**, 369–383.

Block, J., & Martin, B.
Predicting the behavior of children under frustration. *Journal of

Abnormal and Social Psychology, 1955, **51**, 281–285.

Boehm, L., & Nass, M. L.
Social class differences in conscience development. *Child Development,* 1962, **33**, 565–574.

Bostow, D. E., & Bailey, J. B.
Modification of severe disruptive and aggressive behavior using brief timeout and reinforcement procedures. *Journal of Applied Behavior Analysis,* 1969, **2**, 31–37.

Brown, G. D., & Tyler, V. O., Jr.
Timeout from reinforcement: A technique for dethroning the "Duke" of an institutionalized delinquent group. *Journal of Child Psychology and Psychiatry,* 1968, **9**, 203–211.

Brown, J. L.
Prognosis from symptoms of preschool children with atypical development. *American Journal of Orthopsychiatry,* 1960, **30**, 382–391.

Brown, P., & Elliott, R.
Control of aggression in a nursery school class. *Journal of Experimental Child Psychology,* 1965, **2**, 103–107.

Brown, R. A., Pace, Z. S., & Becker, W. C.
Treatment of extreme negativism and autistic behavior in a 6-year-old boy. *Exceptional Children,* 1969, **36**, 115–122.

Browning, R. M.
Effect of irrelevant peripheral visual stimuli on discrimination learning in minimally brain-damaged children. *Journal of Consulting Psychology,* 1967, **31**, 371–376.

Browning, R. M., & Stover, D. O.
Behavior modification in child treatment. Chicago: Aldine-Atherton, 1971.

Bruch, H.
Conceptual confusion in eating disorders. *Journal of Nervous and Mental Diseases,* 1961, **133**, 46–54.

Bruch, H.
Perceptual and conceptual disturbances in anorexia nervosa. *Psychosomatic Medicine*, 1962, **24**, 187–194.

Burchard, J., & Tyler, V. O., Jr.
The modification of delinquent behavior through operant conditioning. *Behaviour Research and Therapy*, 1965, **2**, 245–250.

Buss, A. H.
The psychology of aggression. New York: Wiley, 1961.

Cattell, R. B.
Personality: A systematic theoretical and factual study. New York: McGraw-Hill, 1950.

Cavan, R. S.
Juvenile delinquency: Development—treatment—control. (2nd ed.) Philadelphia: Lippincott, 1962.

Chalfant, J. C., & Scheffelin, M. A.
Central processing dysfunctions in children: A review of research. Bethesda, Md.: U. S. Department of Health, Education, and Welfare, 1969. (NINDS Monograph 9)

Clark, J. P., & Wenninger, E. P.
Socio-economic class and area as correlates of illegal behavior among juveniles. *American Sociological Review*, 1962, **27**, 826–834.

Clausen, J.
Ability structure and subgroups in mental retardation. New York: Spartan Books, 1966.

Clement, P. W., & Milne, D. C.
Group play therapy and tangible reinforcers used to modify the behavior of eight-year-old boys. *Proceedings of the 75th Annual Convention of the American Psychological Association,* 1967, **2**, 241–242.

Clements, S. D.
Minimal brain dysfunction in children. Washington, D. C.: U. S. Department of Health, Education, and Welfare, 1966. (NINDB Monograph 3; USPHS Publication 1415)

Clements, S. D. (Project Director)
Minimal brain dysfunction in children. Washington, D.C.: U.S. Department of Health, Education, and Welfare, 1969. (USPHS Publication 2015)

Cloward, R., & Ohlin, L.
Delinquency and opportunity: A theory of delinquent gangs. Glencoe, Ill.: Free Press, 1960.

Coleman, J. C., & Sandhu, M.
A descriptive-relational study of 364 children referred to a university clinic for learning disorders. *Psychological Reports,* 1967, **20**, 1091–1105.

Compton, R. D.
Changes in enuretics accompanying treatment by the conditioned response technique. *Dissertation Abstracts,* 1968, **28**, (7-A), 2549.

Connerly, R. J.
A comparison of personality characteristics for parents of brain-injured and normal children. *Dissertation Abstracts,* 1967, **28**, 1291–1292.

Conners, C. K.
Symptom patterns in hyperkinetic, neurotic, and normal children. *Child Development,* 1970, **41**, 667–682.

Conners, C. K., Eisenberg, L., & Barcai, A.
Effect of dextroamphetamine on children: Studies on subjects with learning disabilities and school behavior problems. *Archives of General Psychiatry,* 1967, **17**, 478–485.

Cowan, P. A., Hoddinott, B. A., & Wright, B. A.
Compliance and resistance in the conditioning of autistic children: An exploratory study. *Child Development,* 1965, **36**, 913–923.

Cowan, P. A., & Walters, R. H.
Studies of reinforcement of aggression: I. Effects of scheduling. *Child Development,* 1963, **34**, 543–551.

Croxen, M. E., & Lytton, H.
Reading disability and difficulties in finger localization and right-left discrimination. *Developmental Psychology,* 1971, **5**, 256–262.

Davison, G. C.
A social learning therapy programme with an autistic child. *Behaviour Research and Therapy,* 1964, **2**, 149–159.

Davison, G. C.
An intensive long-term social-learning treatment program with an accurately diagnosed autistic child. *Proceedings of the 73rd Annual Convention of the American Psychological Association,* 1965, **1**, 203–204.

Davitz, J. L.
The effects of previous training on postfrustration behavior. *Journal of Abnormal and Social Psychology,* 1952, **47**, 309–315.

DeLeon, G., & Mandell, W.
A comparison of conditioning and psychotherapy in the treatment of functional enuresis. *Journal of Clinical Psychology,* 1966, **22**, 326–330.

DesLauriers, A. M., & Carlson, C.F.
Your child is asleep: Early infantile autism, etiology, treatment, parental influences. Homewood, Ill.: Dorsey, 1969.

Dingman, H. F., & Tarjan, G.
Mental retardation and the normal distribution curve. *American Journal of Mental Deficiency,* 1960, **64**, 991–994.

Dollard, J., Doob, L. W., Miller, N. E., Mowrer, O. H., & Sears, R. R.
Frustration and aggression. New Haven: Yale, 1939.

Doubros, S. G., & Daniels, G. J.
An experimental approach to the reduction of overactive behavior. *Behaviour Research and Therapy,* 1966, **4**, 251–258.

Dreger, R. M., Lewis, P. M., Rich, T. A., Miller, K. S., Reid, M. P., Overlade, D. C., Taffel, C., & Flemming, E. L.
Behavioral classification project. *Journal of Consulting Psychology,* 1964, **28**, 1–13.

Dykman, R. A., Walls, R. C., Suzuki, T., Ackerman, P. T., & Peters, J. E.
Children with learning disabilities: Conditioning, differentiation, and the effect of distraction. *American Journal of Orthopsychiatry,* 1970, **40**, 766–782.

Eaton, L., & Menolascino, F. J.
Psychotic reactions of childhood: A follow-up study. *American Journal of Orthopsychiatry,* 1967, **37**, 521–529.

Eisenberg, L.
The autistic child in adolescence. *American Journal of Psychiatry,* 1956, **112**, 607–612.

Erickson, M. L., & Empey, L. T.
Class position, peers and delinquency. *Sociology and Social Research,* 1965, **49**, 268–282.

Estes, W. K.
Learning theory and mental development. New York: Academic, 1970.

Eysenck, H. J.
The dynamics of anxiety and hysteria. New York: Praeger, 1957.

Eysenck, H. J. (Ed.)
Behavior therapy and the neuroses. New York: Pergamon, 1960.

Eysenck, H. J.
New ways in psychotherapy. *Psychology Today,* 1967, **1**, 39–47.

Ferster, C. B.
Positive reinforcement and behavioral deficits of autistic children. *Child Development,* 1961, **32**, 437–456.

Ferster, C. B.
Arbitrary and natural reinforcement. *Psychological Record,* 1967, **17**, 341–347.

Ferster, C. B., & DeMyer, M. K.
A method for the experimental analysis of the behavior of autistic children. *American Journal of Orthopsychiatry,* 1962, **32**, 89–98.

Fineman, K. R.
An operant conditioning program in a juvenile detention facility. *Psychological Reports,* 1968, **22**, 1119–1120.

Frith, U.
Studies in pattern detection in normal and autistic children : I. Immediate recall of auditory sequences. *Journal of Abnormal Psychology,* 1970, **76**, 413–420.

Funkenstein, D. H., King, S. H., & Drolette, M.E.
Mastery of stress. Cambridge, Mass. : Harvard, 1957.

Gardner, J. M.
Teaching behavior modification to nonprofessionals. *Journal of Applied Behavior Analysis,* 1972, **5**, 517–521.

Garvey, W. P., & Hegrenes, J. R.
Desensitization techniques in the treatment of school phobia. *American Journal of Orthopsychiatry,* 1966, **36**, 147–152.

Gelber, H., & Meyer, V.
Behaviour therapy and encopresis :   The complexities involved in treatment. *Behaviour Research and Therapy,* 1965, **2**, 227–231.

Gelfand, D. M., & Hartman, D. P.
Behavior therapy with children : A review and evaluation of research methodology. *Psychological Bulletin,* 1968, **69**, 204–215.

Gesell, A.
The conditioned reflex and the psychiatry of infancy. *American Journal of Orthopsychiatry,* 1938, **8**, 19–29.

Gewirtz, J. L., & Stingle, K. G.
Learning of generalized imitation as the basis for identification. *Psychological Review,* 1968, **5**, 374–397.

Gilbert, G. M.
A survey of "referral problems" in Metropolitan child guidance centers. *Journal of Clinical Psychology,* 1957, **13**, 37–42.

Giles, D. K., & Wolf, M. M.
Toilet training institutionalized severe retardates : An application of

operant behavior modification techniques. *American Journal of Mental Deficiency,* 1966, **70**, 766–780.

Glueck, S., & Glueck, E.
Unraveling juvenile delinquency. Cambridge, Mass.: Harvard, 1950.

Glueck, S., & Glueck, E.
Predicting delinquency and crime. Cambridge, Mass.: Harvard, 1959.

Glueck, S., & Glueck, E.
Family environment and delinquency. Boston: Houghton Mifflin, 1962.

Goldfarb, W.
Childhood schizophrenia. Cambridge, Mass.: Harvard, 1961.

Goldfarb, W.
Childhood psychosis. In P. H. Mussen (Ed.), *Carmichael's Manual of Child Psychology,* (3rd ed.) Vol. II. New York: Wiley, 1970. Pp. 765–830.

Goldiamond, I., & Dyrud, J. E.
Reading as operant behavior. In J. Money (Ed.), *The disabled reader: Education of the dyslexic child.* Baltimore: Johns Hopkins, 1966. Pp. 93–115.

Goodkin, R.
Some neglected issues in the literature on behavior therapy. *Psychological Reports,* 1967, **20**, 415–420.

Group for the Advancement of Psychiatry.
Psychopathological disorders in childhood: Theoretical considerations and a proposed classification. GAP Report 62, 1966.

Hagen, J. W., Winsberg, B., & Wolff, P.
Cognitive and linguistic deficits in psychotic children. *Child Development,* 1968, **39**, 1103–1117.

Hall, R. V., Cristler, C., Cranston, S. S., & Tucker, B.
Teachers and parents as researchers using multiple baseline designs. *Journal of Applied Behavior Analysis,* 1970, **3**, 247–255.

Hall, R. V., Fox, R., Willard, D., Goldsmith, L., Emerson, M., Owen, M., Davis, F., & Porcia, E.
The teacher as observer and experimenter in the modification of disputing and talking-out behavior. *Journal of Applied Behavior Analysis,* 1971, **4**, 141–149.

Hallsten, E. A., Jr.
Adolescent anorexia nervosa treated by desensitization. *Behaviour Research and Therapy,* 1965, **3**, 87–91.

Haring, N. G., & Bateman, B. D.
Introduction. In *Minimal brain dysfunctions in children.* U. S. Public Health Publication No. 2015. Washington, D. C.: U. S. Department of Health, Education, and Welfare, 1969. Pp. 1–4.

Harris, F. R., Johnston, M. K., Kelley, C. S., & Wolf, M. M.
Effects of positive social reinforcement on regressed crawling of a nursery school child. In L. P. Ullmann, & L. Krasner (Eds.), *Case studies in behavior modification.* New York: Holt, 1965. Pp. 313–319.

Hart, B. M., Allen, K. E., Buell, J. S., Harris, F. B., & Wolf, M. M.
Effects of social reinforcement on operant crying. In L. P. Ullmann & L. Krasner (Eds.), *Case studies in behavior modification.* New York: Holt, 1965. Pp. 320–325.

Hawkins, R. P., Peterson, R. F., Schweid, E., & Bijou, S. W.
Behavior therapy in the home: Amelioration of problem parent-child relations with the parent in a therapeutic role. *Journal of Experimental Child Psychology,* 1966, **4**, 99–107.

Heber, R. F.
A manual on terminology and classification in mental retardation. *American Journal of Mental Deficiency,* 1959, **64**, Monograph supplement (Rev. ed., 1961).

Heller, K. M.
Conceptual sorting and childhood schizophrenia. *Dissertation Abstracts,* 1966, **26**, 6168.

Hermelin, B., & O'Connor, N.
Visual imperception in psychotic children. *British Journal of Psychology,* 1965, **56**, 455–460.

Hermelin, B., & O'Connor, N.
Perceptual and motor discrimination in psychotic and normal children. *Journal of Genetic Psychology*, 1967, **110**, 117-125.

Hess, R. D.
Social class and ethnic influences upon socialization. In P. H. Mussen (Ed.), *Carmichael's Manual of Child Psychology* (3rd ed.) Vol. II. New York: Wiley, 1970. Pp. 457-557.

Hess, R. D., & Shipman, V. C.
Early experience and the socialization of cognitive modes in children. *Child Development,* 1965, **34**, 869–886.

Hess, R. D., & Shipman, V. C.
Cognitive elements in maternal behavior. In J. P. Hill (Ed.), *Minnesota Symposia on Child Psychology*. Vol. I. Minneapolis: University of Minnesota Press, 1967.

Hewett, F. M.
Teaching speech to an autistic child through operant conditioning. *American Journal of Orthopsychiatry*, 1965, **35**, 927–936.

Hewett, F. M., Mayhew, D., & Rabb, E.
An experimental reading program for neurologically impaired, mentally retarded, and severally emotionally disturbed children. *American Journal of Orthopsychiatry,* 1967, **37**, 35–48.

Hewitt, L. E., & Jenkins, R. L.
Fundamental patterns of maladjustment: The dynamics of their origin. Springfield, Ill.: State of Illinois, 1946.

Hill, J. H., Liebert, R. M., & Mott, D. E.
Vicarious extinction of avoidance behavior through films: An initial test. *Psychological Reports,* 1968, **22**, 192.

Hirsch, I. S.
Training mothers in groups as reinforcement therapists for their own children. *Dissertation Abstracts*, 1968, **28** (11-B), 4756.

Hoffman, M. L.
Moral development. In P. H. Mussen (Ed.), *Carmichael's Manual*

of Child Psychology. (3rd ed.) Vol. II. New York: Wiley, 1970. Pp. 261–359.

Hokfelt, B.
Noradrenaline and adrenaline in mammalian tissues. *Acta Physiologica Scandinavica*, 1951, Supplement 92.

Hollenberg, E., & Sperry, M.
Some antecedents of aggression and effects of frustration in doll play. *Journal of Personality,* 1951, **1**, 32–43.

Hops, H., & Walters, R. H.
Studies of reinforcement of aggression: II. Effects of emotionally-arousing antecedent conditions. *Child Development,* 1963, **34**, 553–562.

Hundziak, M., Maurer, R. A., & Watson, L. S., Jr.
Operant conditioning in toilet training or severely mentally retarded boys. *American Journal of Mental Deficiency,* 1965, **70**, 120–124.

Hunt, J. McV.
Intelligence and experience. New York: Ronald, 1961.

Hutt, S. J., Hutt, C., Lee, D., & Ornsted, C.
A behavioural and electroencephalographic study of autistic children. *Journal of Psychiatric Research,* 1965, **3**, 181–197.

Irwin, O. C.
The amount and nature of activities of newborn infants under constant external stimulating conditions during the first ten days of life. *Genetic Psychology Monographs*, 1930, **8**, 1–92.

Ivanov-Smolenski, A. G.
Neurotic behavior and teaching of conditioned reflexes. *American Journal of Psychiatry*, 1927, **7**, 483–488.

Jenkins, R. L., & Hewitt, L.
Types of personality structure encountered in child guidance clinics. *American Journal of Orthopsychiatry*, 1944, **14**, 84–94.

Jensen, G. D., & Womack, M. G.
Operant conditioning techniques applied in the treatment of an

autistic child. *American Journal of Orthopsychiatry*, 1967, **37**, 30–34.

Jones, H. G.
The behavioral treatment of enuresis nocturna. In H. J. Eysenck (Ed.), *Behaviour therapy and the neuroses*. London; Pergamon, 1960. Pp. 377–403.

Jones, M. C.
A laboratory study of fear: The case of Peter. *Pediatrics Seminar*, 1924, **31**, 308–315. (a)

Jones, M. C.
The elimination of children's fears. *Journal of Experimental Psychology*, 1924, **7**, 383–390. (b)

Johnson, S. M., & Brown, R. A.
Producing behavior change in parents of disturbed children. *Journal of Child Psychology and Psychiatry*, 1969, **10**, 107–121.

Kanfer, F. H., & Phillips, J. S.
Behavior therapy: A panacea for all ills or a passing fancy? *Archives of General Psychiatry*, 1966, **15**, 114–128.

Kanner, L.
Autistic disturbances of affective contact. *Nervous Child*, 1943, **2**, 217–240.

Kanner, L.
The specificity of early infantile autism. *Zeitschrift für Kinderpsychiatrie*, 1958, **25**, 108–113.

Kaspar, J. C., Millichap, J. G., Backus, R., Child, D., & Schulman, J. L.
A study of the relationship between neurological evidence of brain damage in children and activity and distractibility. *Journal of Consulting and Clinical Psychology*, 1971, **36**, 329–337.

Katkin, E. S., & Murray, E. N.
Instrumental conditioning of autonomically mediated behavior: Theoretical and methodological issues. *Psychological Bulletin*, 1968, **70**, 52–68.

Kennedy, W. A.
School phobia: Rapid treatment of fifty cases. *Journal of Abnormal Psychology*, 1965, **70**, 285–289.

Kephart, N. C.
The slow learner in the classroom. Columbus, Ohio: Merrill, 1960.

Kessen, W., & Mandler, G.
Anxiety, pain and the inhibition of distress. *Psychological Review,* 1961, **68**, 396–404.

Kessler, J. W.
Psychopathology of childhood. Englewood Cliffs, N. J.: Prentice-Hall, 1966.

King, D. L.
A review and interpretation of some aspects of the infant-mother relationship in mammals and birds. *Psychological Bulletin*, 1966, **65**, 143–155.

Kingsley, R. F.
Associative learning ability in educable mentally retarded children. *American Journal of Mental Deficiency*, 1968, **73**, 5–8.

Klebanoff, L. B.
Parents of schizophrenic children: I. Parental attitudes of mothers of schizophrenic, brain-injured and retarded, and normal children. *American Journal of Orthopsychiatry*, 1959, **29**, 445–454.

Koegel, R. L., & Covert, A.
The relationship of self-stimulation to learning in autistic children. *Journal of Applied Behavior Analysis,* 1972, **5**, 381-387.

Kohlberg, L.
Moral development and identification. In H. W. Stevenson, J. Kagan, & C. Spiker (Eds.), *Child Psychology, The 62nd Yearbook of the National Society for the Study of Education.* Chicago: National Society for the Study of Education, 1963. Pp. 277–332.

Kohlberg, L.
Development of moral character and moral ideology. In M. Hoffman

& L. W. Hoffman (Eds.), *Review of child development research.* Vol. 1. New York: Russell Sage, 1964. Pp. 383–431.

Kohlenberg, R. J.
The punishment of persistent vomiting. *Journal of Applied Behavior Analysis,* 1970, **3**, 241–245.

Kohn, M.
Congruent competence and symptom factors in the preschool child. Paper presented at the meeting of the American Psychological Association, Washington, D. C., September, 1969.

Krasnogorski, N. I.
The conditioned reflex and children's neuroses. *American Journal of Diseases of Children,* 1925, **30**, 753–768.

Lal, H., & Lindsley, O. R.
Therapy of chronic constipation in a young child by rearranging social contingencies. *Behaviour Research and Therapy,* 1968, **6**, 484–485.

Lang, P. J., Lazovik, A. D., & Reynolds, D. J.
Desensitization, suggestibility, and pseudotherapy. *Journal of Abnormal Psychology,* 1965, **70**, 395–402.

Lang, P. J., & Melamed, B. G.
Avoidance conditioning therapy of an infant with chronic ruminative vomiting: Case report. *Journal of Abnormal Psychology,* 1969, **74**, 1–8.

Lapouse, R., & Monk, M. A.
Fears and worries in a representative sample of children. *American Journal of Orthopsychiatry,* 1959, **29**, 803–818.

Lapouse, R., & Monk, M. A.
Behavior deviations in a representative sample of children: Variation by sex, age, race, social class and family size. *American Journal of Orthopsychiatry,* 1964, **34**, 436–446.

Lazarus, A. A.
The elimination of children's phobias by deconditioning. *Medical Proceedings of South Africa,* 1959, **5**, 261–265.

Lazarus, A. A., & Abramovitz, A.
The use of "emotive imagery" in the treatment of children's phobias. In L. P. Ullmann, & L. Krasner (Eds.), *Case studies in behavior modification.* New York: Holt, 1965. Pp. 300–304.

Lazarus, A. A., Davison, G. C., & Polefka, D. A.
Classical and operant factors in the treatment of a school phobia. *Journal of Abnormal Psychology,* 1965, **70**, 225–229.

Leff, R.
Behavior modification and the psychoses of childhood: A review. *Psychological Bulletin,* 1968, **69**, 396–409.

Leitenberg, H., Agras, S., Butz, R., & Wincze, J.
Relationship between heart rate and behavioral change during the treatment of phobias. *Journal of Abnormal Psychology,* 1971, **78**, 59–68.

Leitenberg, H., Agras, W. S., & Thomson, L. E.
A sequential analysis of the effect of selective positive reinforcement in modifying anorexia nervosa. *Behaviour Research and Therapy,* 1968, **6**, 211–218.

Levitt, E. E.
The results of psychotherapy with children: An evaluation. *Journal of Consulting Psychology,* 1957, **21**, 189–196.

Levitt, E. E.
Psychotherapy with children: A further evaluation. *Behaviour Research and Therapy,* 1963, **1**, 45–51.

Liebert, R. M., Hanratty, M., & Hill, J. H.
Effects of rule structure and training method on the adoption of a self-imposed standard. *Child Development,* 1969, **40**, 93–101.

Liebert, R. M., & Ora, J. P., Jr.
Children's adoption of self-reward patterns: Incentive level and method of transmission. *Child Development,* 1968, **39**, 537–544.

Lipton, E. L., Steinschneider, A., & Richmond, J. B.
Psychophysiologic disorders in children. In L. W. Hoffman & M. L. Hoffman (Eds.), *Review of child development research.* Vol. 2. New York: Russell Sage, 1966. Pp. 169–220.

Lore, R. K.
Palmar sweating and transitory anxieties in children. *Child Development*, 1966, **37**, 115–123.

Lorr, M., & Jenkins, R. L.
Patterns of maladjustment in children. *Journal of Clinical Psychology*, 1953, **9**, 16–23.

Lovaas, O. I.
Effect of exposure to symbolic aggression on aggressive behavior. *Child Development*, 1961, **32**, 37–44. (a)

Lovaas, O. I.
Interaction between verbal and nonverbal behavior. *Child Development*, 1961, **32**, 329–336. (b)

Lovaas, O. I.
A program for the establishment of speech in psychotic children. In J. K. Wing (Ed.), *Early childhood autism*. New York: Pergamon, 1966. Pp. 115–144.

Lovaas, O. I., Freitag, G., Gold, V. J., & Kassorla, I. C.
Experimental studies in childhood schizophrenia: Analysis of self-destructive behavior. *Journal of Experimental Child Psychology*, 1965, **2**, 67–84.

Lovaas, O. I., Freitag, G., Kinder, M. I., Rubenstein, B. D., Schaeffer, B., & Simmons, J. Q.
Establishment of social reinforcers in two schizophrenic children on the basis of food. *Journal of Experimental Child Psychology*, 1966, **4**, 109–125.

Lovaas, O. I., Freitas, L., Nelson, K., & Whalen, C.
The establishment of imitation and its use for the development of complex behavior in schizophrenic children. *Behaviour Research and Therapy*, 1967, **5**, 171–181.

Lovaas, O. I., Koegel, R., Simmons, J. Q., & Long, J. S.
Some generalization and follow-up measures on autistic children in behavior therapy. *Journal of Applied Behavior Analysis*, 1973, **6**, 131-166.

Lovaas, O. I., Schaeffer, B., & Simmons, J. Q.
Building social behavior in autistic children by use of electric shock. *Journal of Experimental Research in Personality*, 1965, **1**, 99–109.

Lovaas, O. I., Schreibman, L., Koegel, R., & Rehm, R.
Selective responding by autistic children to multiple sensory input. *Journal of Abnormal Psychology*, 1971, **77**, 211-222.

Lovibond, S. H.
The mechanism of conditioning treatment of enuresis. *Behaviour Research and Therapy*, 1963, **1**, 17–21.

Lovibond, S. H.
Conditioning and enuresis. New York: Pergamon, 1964.

Lovitt, T. C.
Assessment of children with learning disabilities. *Exceptional Children*, 1967, **34**, 233–239.

Luckey, R. E., Watson, C. M., & Musick, J. K.
Aversive conditioning as a means of inhibiting vomiting and rumination. *American Journal of Mental Deficiency*, 1968, **73**, 139–142.

McCarthy, J. J., & McCarthy, J. F.
Learning disabilities. Boston: Allyn and Bacon, 1969.

McCord, W., & McCord, J.
Origins of crime: A new evaluation of the Cambridge-Somerville Youth Study. New York: Columbia, 1959.

McDermott, J. F., Jr., Harrison, S. I., Schrager, J., Lindy, J., & Killins, E.
Social class and mental illness in children: The question of childhood psychosis. *American Journal of Orthopsychiatry*, 1967, **37**, 548–557.

McLeod, J. M.
An investigation of the Frostig program in teaching children with extreme learning problems. *Dissertation Abstracts*, 1967, **28**, 1303.

Mahler, M. S.
On child psychosis and schizophrenia: Autistic and symbiotic infantile psychosis. *Psychoanalytic Study of the Child*, 1952, **7**, 286–305.

Mallick, S. K., & McCandless, B. R.
A study of catharsis of aggression. *Journal of Personality and Social Psychology*, 1966, **4**, 591–596.

Marr, J. N., Miller, E. R., & Straub, R. R.
Operant conditioning of attention with a psychotic girl. *Behavior Research and Therapy*, 1966, **4**, 85–87.

Martin, B.
The assessment of anxiety by physiological behavioral measures. *Psychological Bulletin*, 1961, **58**, 234–255.

Masland, R. L., Sarason, S. B., & Gladwin, T.
Mental subnormality. New York: Basic Books, 1958.

Masters, J. C., & Miller, D. E.
Early infantile autism: A methodological critique. *Journal of Abnormal Psychology*, 1970, **75**, 342–343.

Mednick, S. A.
Breakdown in individuals at high risk for schizophrenia: possible predispositional perinatal factors. *Mental Hygiene*, 1970, **54**, 50–63.

Mednick, S. A., & Schulsinger, F.
Some premorbid characteristics related to breakdown in children with schizophrenic mothers. *Journal of Psychiatric Research*, 1968, **6**, 267–291.

Metz, J. R.
Conditioning generalized imitation in autistic children. *Journal of Experimental Child Psychology*, 1965, **2**, 389–399.

Metz, J. R.
Stimulation level preferences of autistic children. *Journal of Abnormal Psychology*, 1967, **72**, 529–535.

Miller, L. C.
Dimensions of psychopathology in middle childhood. *Psychological Reports*, 1967, **21**, 897–903. (a)

Miller, L. C.
Louisville Behavior Check List for males, 6-12 years of age. *Psychological Reports*, 1967, **21**, 885–896. (b)

Miller, L. C.
Pittsburgh Adjustment Survey Scales : A cross validation and normative study. Unpublished manuscript, University of Louisville, 1968.

Miller, L. C., Hampe, E., Barrett, C. L., & Noble, H.
Children's deviant behavior within the general population. *Journal of Consulting and Clinical Psychology*, 1971, **37**, 16–22.

Miller, W. B.
Lower class culture as a generating milieu of gang delinquency. *Journal of Social Issues*, 1958, **14**, 5–19.

Mischel, W.
Preference for delayed reinforcement and social responsibility. *Journal of Abnormal and Social Psychology*, 1961, **62**, 1–7.

Mischel, W.
Theory and research on the antecedents of self-imposed delay or reward. In B. A. Maher (Ed.), *Progress in experimental personality research*. Vol. 3. New York : Academic, 1966. Pp. 85–132.

Mischel, W.
Personality and assessment. New York : Wiley, 1968.

Mischel, W., & Gilligan, C.
Delay of gratification, motivation for the prohibited gratification, and responses to temptation. *Journal of Abnormal and Social Psychology*, 1964, **69**, 411–417.

Mischel, W., & Liebert, R. M.
Effects of discrepancies between observed and imposed reward criteria on their acquisition and transmission. *Journal of Personality and Social Psychology*, 1966, **3**, 45–53.

Mischel, W., & Liebert, R. M.
The role of power in the adoption of self-reward patterns. *Child Development*, 1967, **38**, 673–683.

Mischel, W., & Metzner, R.
Preference for delayed reward as a function of age, intelligence, and length of delay interval. *Journal of Abnormal and Social Psychology*, 1962, **64**, 425–431.

Morgan, S. B.
Responsiveness to stimulus novelty and complexity in mild, moderate and severe retardates. *American Journal of Mental Deficiency*, 1969, **74**, 32–38.

Mostofsky, D. I.
Attention: Contemporary theory and analysis. New York: Appleton-Century-Crofts, 1970.

Mowrer, O. H.
Two-factor learning theory: Summary and comment. *Psychological Review*, 1951, **58**, 350–354.

Mowrer, O. H., & Aiken, E. G.
Contiguity vs. drive reduction in conditioned fear: Temporal variations in conditioned and unconditioned stimulus. *American Journal of Psychology*, 1954, **67**, 26–38.

Mowrer, O. H., & Mowrer, W. M.
Enuresis: A method for its study and treatment. *American Journal of Orthopsychiatry*, 1938, **8**, 436–459.

Neale, D. H.
Behaviour therapy and encopresis in children. *Behaviour Research and Therapy*, 1963, **1**, 139–149.

Nisbett, R. E., & Valins, S.
Perceiving the causes of one's own behavior. New York: General Learning Press, 1971.

Nolan, J. D., Mattis, P. R., & Holliday, W. C.
Long-term effects of behavior therapy: A 12-month follow-up. *Journal of Abnormal Psychology*, 1970, **76**, 88–92.

Novick, J.
Symptomatic treatment of acquired and persistent enuresis. *Journal of Abnormal Psychology*, 1966, **71**, 363–368.

Novick, J., Rosenfeld, E., Bloch, D. A., & Dawson, D.
Ascertaining deviant behavior in children. *Journal of Consulting Psychology*, 1966, **30**, 230–238.

Nye, F. I.
Family relationships and juvenile delinquency. New York: Wiley, 1958.

Nye, F. I., Short, J. F., & Olson, V. J.
Socioeconomic status and delinquent behavior. *American Journal of Sociology,* 1958, **63**, 381–389.

O'Leary, K. D., & Becker, W. C.
Behavior modification of an adjustment class: A token reinforcement program. *Exceptional Children,* 1967, **33**, 637–642.

O'Leary, K. D., Becker, W. C., Evans, M. B., & Saudargas, R. A.
A token reinforcement program in a public school: A replication and systematic analysis. *Journal of Applied Behavior Analysis,* 1969, **2,** 3–13.

O'Leary, K. D., O'Leary, S., & Becker, W. C.
Modification of a deviant sibling interaction pattern in the home. *Behaviour Research and Therapy,* 1967, **5**, 113–120.

Owen, F. W., Adams, P. A., Forrest, T., Stolz, L. M., & Fisher, S.
Learning disorders in children: sibling studies. *Monographs of the Society for Research in Child Development,* 1971, **36**, 4 (Whole No. 144).

Palermo, D. S., Castaneda, A., & McCandless, B. R.
The relationship of anxiety in children to performance in a complex learning task. *Child Development,* 1956, **27**, 333–337.

Parton, D. A.
The study of aggression in boys with an operant device. *Journal of Experimental Child Psychology,* 1964, **1**, 79–80.

Patterson, G. R.
An empirical approach to the classification of disturbed children. *Journal of Clinical Psychology,* 1964, **20**, 326–337.

Patterson, G. R.
An application of conditioning techniques to the control of a hyperactive child. In L. Ullmann & L. Krasner (Eds.), *Case studies in behavior modification.* New York: Holt, 1965. Pp. 370–375.

Patterson, G. R., & Brodsky, G.
A behavior modification programme for a child with multiple problem behaviors. *Journal of Child Psychology and Psychiatry*, 1966, **7**, 277–295.

Patterson, G. R., Helper, M. E., & Wilcott, R. C.
Anxiety and verbal conditioning in children. *Child Development*, 1960, **31**, 101–108.

Patterson, G. R., Jones, R., Whittier, J., & Wright, M. A.
A behaviour modification technique for the hyperactive child. *Behaviour Research and Therapy*, 1965, **2**, 217–226.

Patterson, G. R., Littman, R. A., & Bricker, W.
Assertive behavior in children : A step toward a theory of aggression. *Monographs of the Society for Research in Child Development*, 1967, **32**, 5 (Whole No. 113).

Patterson, G. R., Ray, R. S., & Shaw, D. A.
Direct intervention in families of deviant children. *Oregon Research Institute Research Bulletin*, 1968, **8**, No. 9.

Paul, G. L.
Insight vs. desensitization in psychotherapy. Stanford, Calif.: Stanford, 1966.

Paul, G. L.
Insight versus desensitization in psychotherapy two years after termination. *Journal of Consulting Psychology*, 1967, **31**, 333–348. (a)

Paul, G. L.
Strategy of outcome research in psychotherapy. *Journal of Consulting Psychology*, 1967, **31**, 109–118. (b)

Paul, G. L., & Shannon, D. T.
Treatment of anxiety through systematic desensitization in therapy groups. *Journal of Abnormal Psychology*, 1966, **71**, 124–135.

Penrose, L. S.
The biology of mental defect. London : Sidgwick & Jackson, 1963.

Peterson, D. R.
Behavior problems of middle childhood. *Journal of Consulting*

Psychology, 1961, **25**, 205–209.

Phillips, E. L., Phillips, E. A., Fixsen, D. L., & Wolf, M. M.
Achievement Place: Modification of the behaviors of pre-delinquent boys with a token economy. *Journal of Applied Behavior Analysis*, 1971, **4**, 45–59.

Powers, E., & Witmer, H.
An experiment in the prevention of delinquency: The Cambridge-Somerville youth study. New York: Columbia, 1951.

Premack, D.
Toward empirical behavior laws: I. Positive reinforcement. *Psychological Review*, 1959, **66**, 219–233.

Purcell, K.
Distinctions between subgroups of asthmatic children: Children's perceptions of events associated with asthma. *Pediatrics*, 1963, **31**, 486–494.

Purcell, K., Brady, K., Chai, H., Muser, J., Molk, L., Gordon, N., & Means, J.
The effect on asthma in children of experimental separation from the family. *Psychosomatic Medicine*, 1969, **31**, 144–164.

Rescorla, R. A., & Solomon, R. L.
Two-process learning theory: Relationships between Pavlovian conditioning and instrumental learning. *Psychological Review*, 1967, **74**, 151–182.

Richmond, J., & Lustman, S.
Autonomic function in the neonate: I. Implications for psychosomatic theory. *Psychosomatic Medicine*, 1955, **17**, 269–275.

Rickard, H. C., & Mundy, M. B.
Direct manipulation of stuttering behavior: An experimental-clinical approach. In L. P. Ullmann & L. Krasner (Eds.), *Case studies in behavior modification*. New York: Holt, 1965. Pp. 268–275.

Rimland, B.
Infantile autism: The syndrome and its implications for a neural theory of behavior. New York: Appleton-Century-Crofts, 1964.

Risley, T. R.
The effects and side effects of punishing the autistic behaviors of a deviant child. *Journal of Applied Behavior Analysis*, 1968, **1**, 21–34.

Risley, T., & Wolf, M.
Establishing functional speech in echolalic children. *Behaviour Research and Therapy*, 1967, **5**, 73–88.

Ritter, B.
The group desensitization of children's snake phobias using vicarious and contact desensitization procedures. *Behaviour Research and Therapy*, 1968, **6**, 1–6.

Ritvo, E. R., Ornitz, E. M., & LaFranchi, S.
Frequency of repetitive behaviors in early infantile autism and its variants. *Archives of General Psychiatry*, 1968, **19**, 341–347.

Robbins, L. C.
The accuracy of parental recall of child development and of child rearing practices. *Journal of Abnormal and Social Psychology*, 1963, **66**, 261–270.

Roberts, A. H., & Erikson, R. V.
Delay of gratification, Porteus Maze Test performance, and behavioral adjustment in a delinquent group. *Journal of Abnormal Psychology*, 1968, **73**, 449–453.

Robinson, H. B., & Robinson, N. M.
The mentally retarded child: A psychological approach. New York: McGraw-Hill, 1965.

Roos, P., & Oliver, M.
Evaluation of operant conditioning with institutionalized retarded children. *American Journal of Mental Deficiency*, 1969, **74**, 325–330.

Ross, A. O.
A schizophrenic child and his mother. *Journal of Abnormal and Social Psychology*, 1955, **51**, 133–139.

Ross, A. O.
The practice of clinical child psychology. New York: Grune & Stratton, 1959.

Ross, A. O.
The issue of normality in clinical child psychology. *Mental Hygiene*, 1963, **47**, 267–272.

Ross, A. O.
Learning theory and therapy with children. *Psychotherapy: Theory, Research and Practice*, 1964, **1**, 102–108. (a)

Ross, A. O.
The exceptional child in the family. New York: Grune & Stratton, 1964. (b)

Ross, A. O.
Learning difficulties of children: Dysfunctions, disorders, disabilities. *Journal of School Psychology*, 1967, **5**, 82–92. (a)

Ross, A. O.
Review of J. W. Kessler, Psychopathology of childhood. *Contemporary Psychology*, 1967, **12**, 418–419. (b)

Ross, A. O.
The application of behavior principles in therapeutic education, *The Journal of Special Education*, 1967, **1**, 275–286. (c)

Ross, A. O., Lacey, H. M., & Parton, D. A.
The development of a behavior checklist for boys. *Child Development*, 1965, **36**, 1013–1027.

Ruebush, B. K.
Anxiety. In H. W. Stevenson, J. Kagan, & C. Spiker (Eds.), *Child Psychology, The 62nd Yearbook of the National Society for the Study of Education.* Chicago: National Society for the Study of Education, 1963, Pp. 460–516.

Rutter, M., Greefeld, D., & Lockyer, L.
A five- to fifteen-year follow-up study of infantile psychosis: II. Social and behavioural outcome. *British Journal of Psychiatry*, 1967, **113**, 1183–1199.

Rutter, M., & Lockyer, L.
A five- to fifteen-year follow-up study of infantile psychosis: I. De-

scription of sample. *British Journal of Psychiatry,* 1967, **113,** 1169–1182.

Sarason, S., & Gladwin, T.
Psychological and cultural problems in mental subnormals : A review of research. *Genetic Psychology Monographs,* 1958, **57,** 3–290.

Schachter, J.
Pain, fear, and anger in hypertensives and normatensives. *Psychosomatic Medicine,* 1957, **19,** 17–29.

Schachter, S., & Singer, J. E.
Cognitive, social and physiological determinants of emotional state. *Psychological Review,* 1962, **49,** 379–399.

Schaefer, E. S.
Converging conceptual models for maternal behavior and for child behavior. In J. C. Glidewell (Ed.), *Parental attitudes and child behavior.* Springfield, Ill.: Charles C. Thomas, 1961. Pp. 124–146.

Schaefer, E. S., & Bayley, N.
Maternal behavior, child behavior, and their intercorrelations from infancy through adolescence. *Monographs of the Society for Research in Child Development,* 1963, **28,** 3 (Whole No. 87).

Schaefer, H. H.
Self-injurious behavior: Shaping "head-banging" in monkeys. *Journal of Applied Behavior Analysis,* 1970, **3,** 111–116.

Schell, R. E., Stark, J., & Giddan, J. J.
Development of language behavior in an autistic child. *Journal of Speech and Hearing Disorders,* 1967, **32,** 51–64.

Schlichter, K. J., & Ratliff, R. G.
Discrimination learning in juvenile delinquents. *Journal of Abnormal Psychology,* 1971, **77,** 46–48.

Schopler, E.
The development of body image and symbol formation through bodily contact with an autistic child. *Journal of Child Psychology and Psychiatry,* 1962, **3,** 191–202.

Schopler, E.
Early infantile autism and receptor processes. *Archives of General Psychiatry,* 1965, **13**, 327–335.

Schopler, E.
Visual versus tactual receptor preference in normal and schizophrenic children. *Journal of Abnormal Psychology,* 1966, **71**, 108–114.

Schwitzgebel, R.
Street-corner research: An experimental approach to the juvenile delinquent. Cambridge, Mass.: Harvard, 1964.

Schwitzgebel, R.
Short-term operant conditioning of adolescent offenders on socially relevant variables. *Journal of Abnormal Psychology,* 1967, **72**, 134–142.

Shepherd, D. M., & West, G. B.
Methylation in the suprarenal medulla. *Journal of Pharmacy and Pharmacology,* 1951, **3**, 382–383.

Shirley, M. M.
The first two years, a study of twenty-five babies: Vol. III. Personality manifestations. *Institute of Child Welfare Monograph Series,* No. 8. Minneapolis: University of Minnesota Press, 1933.

Shodell, M. J.
Personalities of mothers of nonverbal and verbal schizophrenic children. *Dissertation Abstracts,* 1967, **28**, 1175.

Short, J. F., Jr.
Juvenile delinquency: The sociocultural context. In L. W. Hoffman & M. L. Hoffman (Eds.), *Review of child development research.* Vol. 2. New York: Russell Sage, 1966. Pp. 423–468.

Short, J. F., & Strodtbeck, F. L.
Group process and gang delinquency. Chicago: University of Chicago Press, 1965.

Sibley, S. A.
Reading rate and accuracy of retarded readers as a function of fixed-

ratio schedules of conditioned reinforcement. *Dissertation Abstracts*, 1967, **27**, 4134–4135.

Skinner, B. F.
The behavior of organisms: An experimental analysis. New York: Appleton-Century-Crofts, 1938.

Skinner, B. F.
Science and human behavior. New York: Macmillan, 1953.

Skinner, B. F.
Verbal behavior. New York: Appleton-Century-Crofts, 1957.

Sloat, S. C.
Child rearing practices in childhood schizophrenia: A comparison of ten schizophrenic children and their non-psychotic siblings. *Dissertation Abstracts*, 1966, **27**, 1296–1297.

Smith, R. E., & Sharpe, T. M.
Treatment of a school phobia with implosive therapy. *Journal of Consulting and Clinical Psychology*, 1970, **35**, 239–243.

Solomon, R. L., & Brush, E. S.
Experimentally derived conceptions of anxiety and aversion. In M. R. Jones (Ed.), *Nebraska symposium on motivation*. Lincoln, Neb. : University of Nebraska Press, 1956. Pp. 212–305.

Staats, A. W., & Butterfield, W. H.
Treatment of nonreading in a culturally deprived juvenile delinquent: An application of reinforcement principles. *Child Development*, 1965, **36**, 925–942.

Staats, A. W., Minke, K. A., Goodwin, W., & Landeen, J.
Cognitive behavior modification: "Motivated learning" reading treatment with subprofessional therapy-technicians. *Behaviour Research and Therapy*, 1967, **5**, 283–299.

Stampfl, T. G., & Levis, D. J.
Essentials of Implosive Therapy: A learning-theory-based psychodynamic behavioral therapy. *Journal of Abnormal Psychology*, 1967, **72**, 496–503.

Steisel, I. M., Friedman, C. J., & Wood, A. C., Jr.
Interaction patterns in children with phenylketonuria. *Journal of Consulting Psychology,* 1967, **31**, 162–168.

Stover, D. O., & Giebink, J. W.
Inter-judge reliability of the Pittsburgh Adjustment Survey Scales. *Psychological Reports,* 1967, **21**, 845–848.

Straughan, J. H.
Treatment with child and mother in the playroom. *Behaviour Research and Therapy,* 1964, **2**, 37–41.

Talbot, M.
Panic in school phobia. *American Journal of Orthopsychiatry,* 1957, **27**, 286–296.

Tasto, D. L.
Systematic desensitization, muscle relaxation and visual imagery in the counterconditioning of a four-year-old phobic child. *Behaviour Research and Therapy,* 1969, **7**, 409–411.

Tate, B. G., & Baroff, G. S.
Aversive control of self-injurious behavior in a psychotic boy. *Behaviour Research and Therapy,* 1966, **4**, 281–287.

Tharp, R. G., & Wetzel, R. J.
Behavior modification in the natural environment. New York: Academic, 1969.

Thomas, A., Chess, S., & Birch, H. G.
Temperament and behavior disorders in children. New York: New York University Press, 1968.

Thomas, A., Chess, S., Birch, H. G., Hertzig, M. E., & Korn, S.
Behavioral individuality in early childhood. New York: New York University Press, 1963.

Thomas, D. R., Becker, W. C., & Armstrong, M.
Production and elimination of disruptive classroom behavior by systematically varying teacher's behavior. *Journal of Applied Behavior Analysis,* 1968, **1**, 35–45.

Toby, J.
An evaluation of early identification and intensive treatment programs for pre-delinquents. *Social Problems*, 1965, **13**, 160–175.

Turnbull, J. W.
Asthma conceived as a learned response. *Journal of Psychosomatic Research*, 1962, **6**, 59–70.

Turner, R. K., Young, G. C., & Rachman, S.
Treatment of nocturnal enuresis by conditioning technique. *Behaviour Research and Therapy*, 1970, **8**, 367–381.

Turnure, J., & Zigler, E.
Outer-directedness in the problem solving of normal and retarded children. *Journal of Abnormal and Social Psychology*, 1964, **69**, 427–436.

Tyler, V. O., Jr., & Brown, G. D.
The use of swift, brief isolation as a group control device for institutionalized delinquents. *Behaviour Research and Therapy*, 1967, **5**, 1–9.

Tyler, V. O., Jr., & Brown, G. D.
Token reinforcement of academic performance with institutionalized delinquent boys. *Journal of Educational Psychology*, 1968, **59**, 164–168.

Ullmann, L. P., & Krasner, L.
A psychological approach to abnormal behavior. Englewood Cliffs, N. J.: Prentice-Hall, 1969.

Valins, S.
Emotionality and information concerning internal reactions. *Journal of Personality and Social Psychology*, 1967, **6**, 458–463.

Wahler, R. G.
Oppositional children: A quest for parental reinforcement control. *Journal of Applied Behavior Analysis*, 1969, **2**, 159–170.

Wahler, R. G., Winkel, G. H., Peterson, R. F., & Morrison, D. C.
Mothers as behavior therapists for their own children. *Behaviour Research and Therapy*, 1965, **3**, 113–124.

Walder, L. O., Abelson, R. P., Eron, L. D., Banta, T. J., & Laulicht, J. H.
Development of a peer-rating measure of aggression. *Psychological Reports*, 1961, **9**, 497–556.

Walters, R. H.
On the high-magnitude theory of aggression. *Child Development,* 1964, **35**, 303–304.

Walters, R. H., & Brown, M.
Studies of reinforcement of aggression : III. Transfer of responses to an interpersonal situation. *Child Development*, 1963, **34**, 563–571.

Walters, R. H., & Brown, M.
A test of the high-magnitude theory of aggression. *Journal of Experimental Child Psychology,* 1964, **1**, 376–387.

Walters, R. H., & Demkow, L. F.
Timing of punishment as a determinant of response inhibition. *Child Development,* 1963, **34**, 207–214.

Ward, A. J.
Early infantile autism: Diagnosis, etiology, and treatment. *Psychological Bulletin,* 1970, **73**, 350–362.

Watson, J. B., & Raynor, R.
Conditioned emotional reactions. *Journal of Experimental Psychology,* 1920, **3**, 1–14.

Wechsler, D.
Wechsler Intelligence Scale for Children. New York: Psychological Corporation, 1949.

Wenar, C.
The reliability of mothers' histories. *Child Development,* 1961, **32**, 491–500.

Werry, J. S.
The conditioning treatment of enuresis. *American Journal of Psychiatry,* 1966, **123**, 226–229.

Werry, J. S., & Quay, H. C.
The prevalence of behavior symptoms in younger elementary

school children. *American Journal of Orthopsychiatry,* 1971, **41**, 136–143.

Wetzel, R.
Use of behavioral techniques in a case of compulsive stealing. *Journal of Consulting Psychology,* 1966, **30**, 367–374.

Wetzel, R. J., Baker, J., Roney, M., & Martin, M.
Outpatient treatment of autistic behavior. *Behaviour Research and Therapy,* 1966, **4**, 169–177.

Wing, J. E. (Ed.)
Early childhood autism: Clinical, educational, and social aspects. New York: Pergamon, 1966.

Wolf, M., & Risley, T.
Analysis and modification of deviant child behavior. Paper presented at the meeting of the American Psychological Association, Washington, D. C., September, 1967.

Wolf, M., Risley, T., Johnston, M., Harris, F., & Allen, E.
Application of operant conditioning procedures to the behavior problems of an autistic child: A follow-up and extension. *Behaviour Research and Therapy,* 1967, **5**, 103–111.

Wolf, M. M., Risley, T., & Mees, H. L.
Application of operant conditioning procedures to the behavior problems of an autistic child. *Behaviour Research and Therapy,* 1964, **1**, 305–312.

Wolff, W. M., & Morris, L. A.
Intellectual and personality characteristics of parents of autistic children. *Journal of Abnormal Psychology,* 1971, **77**, 155–161.

Wolpe, J.
Psychotherapy by reciprocal inhibition. Stanford, Calif.,: Stanford, 1958.

Wolpe, J.
The practice of behavior therapy. New York: Pergamon, 1969.

Yarrow, M. R., Waxler, C. Z., & Scott, P. M.
Child effects on adult behavior. *Developmental Psychology,* 1971, **5**, 300–311.

Zaslow, R. W., & Breger, L.
A theory and treatment of autism. In L. Breger (Ed.), *Clinical-cognitive Psychology: Models and integrations.* Englewood Cliffs, N. J.: Prentice-Hall, 1969, Pp. 246–291.

Zeaman, D., & House B. J.
The role of attention in retardate discrimination learning. In N. R. Ellis (Ed.), *Handbook of mental deficiency.* New York: McGraw-Hill, 1963. Pp. 159–223.

Zeilberger, J., Sampen, S. E., & Sloane, H. N., Jr.
Modification of a child's problem behaviors in the home with the mother as therapist. *Journal of Applied Behavior Analysis,* 1968, **1**, 47–53.

Zigler, E.
Developmental versus difference theories of mental retardation and the problem of motivation. *American Journal of Mental Deficiency,* 1960, **73**, 536–556.

Zigler, E.
Mental retardation: Current issues and approaches. In L. W. Hoffman and M. L. Hoffman (Eds.), *Review of child development research.* Vol. 2. New York: Russell Sage, 1966. Pp. 107–168. (a)

Zigler, E.
Research on personality structure of the retardate. In N. R. Ellis (Ed.), *International review of research in mental retardation.* Vol. I. New York: Academic, 1966. Pp. 77–108. (b)

Zigler, E.
Familial mental retardation: A continuing dilemma. *Science,* 1967, **155**, 292–298.

Zigler, E., Butterfield, E. C., & Capobianco, F.
Institutionalization and the effectiveness of social reinforcement:

A 5- and 8-year follow-up study. *Developmental Psychology,* 1970, **3**, 255–263.

Zigler, E., & deLabry, J.
Concept-switching in middle-class, lower-class, and retarded children. *Journal of Abnormal and Social Psychology,* 1962, **65**, 267–273.

Zigler, E., & Phillips, L.
Psychiatric diagnosis: A critique. *Journal of Abnormal and Social Psychology,* 1961, **63**, 607–618.

Zigler, E., & Williams, J.
Institutionalization and the effectiveness of social reinforcement: A three-year follow-up study. *Journal of Abnormal and Social Psychology,* 1963, **66**, 197–205.

NAME INDEX

NAME INDEX

SUBJECT INDEX

SUBJECT INDEX